Audiology

An Introduction for Teachers and Other Professionals

MARYANNE TATE MALTBY
AND PAMELA KNIGHT

Routledge
Taylor & Francis Group
LONDON AND NEW YORK

David Fulton Publishers Ltd
2 Park Square, Milton Park, Abingdon, Oxfordshire OX14 4RN
711 Third Avenue, New York, NY 10017

Routledge is an imprint of the Taylor and Francis Group, an informa business

First issued in hardback 2015

First published in Great Britain by David Fulton Publishers 2000

Note: The right of Maryanne Tate Maltby and Pamela Knight to be identified as the authors of this work has been asserted by them in accordance with the Copyright, Designs and Patents Act 1988.

British Library Cataloguing in Publication Data
A catalogue record for this book is available from the British Library.

ISBN 978-1-85346-665-6 (pbk)
ISBN 978-1-138-13751-6 (hbk)

Contents

Foreword

The primary aim of this book is to meet the audiological needs of those studying to become teachers of the deaf, as well as other teachers and professionals working with deaf students and their families. It will also be of interest to anyone new to the field of deafness and deaf education. This book is intended as an introduction to audiology for those who have little or no previous knowledge. It offers a basic knowledge of audiology to a depth required by teachers of the deaf on training courses and also gives enough information to allow the reader access to the more specialised journal articles and textbooks. The book addresses the practical implications of audiological support for deaf pupils both in the home and in the school setting.

Acknowledgements

The authors wish to express their gratitude to the following people for their help: Sue Archbold (Nottingham Cochlear Implant Team) and Louisa Booth (Advanced Bionics) for their most helpful comments with regard to cochlear implants; Nicola Knight for the freehand diagrams and her innovative ideas; David Gaszczyk for the computer drawn diagrams and for helpful comments and suggestions.

Introduction

A firm knowledge of audiology is essential for all those working with deaf and hearing impaired pupils. Audiology is a scientific subject, which is continually developing and changing. It is important that those who are involved with deaf pupils are responsible for their own continuing professional development in this area. This means personally updating their audiological knowledge through courses, current literature, the internet and journal articles, as well as working closely with other professionals, such as educational audiologists and members of the cochlear implant teams. This book is intended to provide a basic knowledge of audiology, as required by teachers of the deaf, speech and language therapists and others, and to give them sufficient knowledge to access more specialised literature.

Teachers of the deaf are specialist teachers, whose firm base in audiological knowledge is a fundamental part of their specialism. They also need to be competent in the practical areas of assessment and the management of amplification systems. The teacher's knowledge of audiology has many implications for their work.

Firstly, they will be a rich source of information about all aspects of deafness for parents, mainstream teachers and others involved in working with deaf children, as well as for deaf children themselves. When working with the parents of young deaf children, teachers need to understand the effect that the initial diagnosis of deafness can have, upon both deaf and hearing families, and be able to discuss all aspects of deafness from an informed and sensitive standpoint.

Secondly they need to be conversant with all audiological assessment procedures and be able to interpret and discuss the implications of test results with parents and subsequently with other teachers. They need to have a clear understanding of the implications of different types and degrees of deafness in social and educational environments.

Thirdly, they need to be conversant with the most appropriate amplification system for the individual child and be able to work in partnership with families and schools on the effective management of hearing aids and the listening environment. They have a role to play in assessing the effectiveness of hearing aids in the 'real world', at home and school, and are in a unique position to report back to the clinic setting on the effectiveness of prescribed hearing aids.

Teachers of the deaf also need to be conversant with the implications of deafness for language development and the curriculum. They have to be able to contribute to individual education programmes (IEP) which are tailored to the needs of each hearing impaired child, whatever the educational setting. The implementation of audiological knowledge and skill with deaf pupils and their families, in the educational and in the home setting, is a fundamental role of the teacher of the deaf.

Where pupils are developing sign language as a first language, the ultimate aim is one of competent sign bilingualism. This means English (or the language of the country) will become their second language. All deaf children have the right to develop competent literacy skills and spoken language skills in their second language. To this end, audiological support will focus on the accurate assessment of deafness, appropriate amplification and acoustic conditions. Input to the development of listening and spoken language skills should be equal with those deaf children with whom an oral approach is being used.

In the context of this book, the authors have not taken a rigid standpoint on the use of the such terms as 'deaf', 'hearing impaired' and 'hearing loss'. Instead they have reflected terminology that is in common use and sometimes the terms are used interchangeably. Generally, the term 'deaf' has been used in relation to losses of a more profound nature and 'hearing impaired' for those of a mild or moderate nature, but no hard and fast rules have been followed.

This book is especially for all those interested in deaf children who do not yet have a theoretical base in audiology. It does not require prior knowledge of audiology but will furnish the basics and allow access to other books and material for those who wish to extend their knowledge further.

Glossary

acoustic conditioning – training a child to respond to a sound (stimulus) by means of a reward.
acoustic energy – sound.
acoustic feedback – unwanted sound which leaks from an amplification system (usually in the form of a high pitched whistle).
acquired deafness – forms of deafness that have been acquired, e.g. through trauma or infection such as otitis media.
audible frequency range – frequencies the human ear is capable of hearing.
audiogram – a graph showing a person's hearing threshold levels.
audiological descriptors – standard terminology used to describe degrees of deafness and the shape of the audiogram.
audiology – the study of all aspects of hearing and hearing loss.
auditory feedback – perception of the speaker's own voice.
auditory information – information gained through hearing.
auditory pathway – channel through which sound travels (outer, middle and inner ear).
auditory processing – interpretation of acoustic information.
bilingual – describes an individual who uses two or more languages in their everyday lives.
binaural hearing – hearing in both ears.
monaural hearing – hearing in one ear only.
unilateral hearing – hearing in one ear only.
British Sign Language (BSL) – the natural language of the adult deaf community in the UK.
cochlear implant – a device implanted into the cochlea, which aims to stimulate the auditory nerve directly to give a sensation of hearing.
component frequencies – tones which make up a specific sound.
conductive hearing loss – deafness associated with problems in the outer and/or middle ear.
congenital hearing loss – this refers to deafness which may be inherited, or due to environmental factors, such as illness during the mother's pregnancy.
first language – a child's first language is normally the language of their home environment and of the wider society in which they live. For

deaf children it is the language they prefer to use, regardless of the home language.

glue ear – a common condition in young children related to infections in the middle ear.

hearing status – this term is used when considering a person or family in terms of whether they are a hearing family, a deaf family or a family with both deaf and hearing members.

mild hearing loss – a hearing loss of between 20 dBHL – 40 dBHL.

moderate hearing loss – a hearing loss of between 41 dBHL – 70 dBHL.

oral method – the method of developing language in deaf children which precludes the use of any form of formalised signs.

oral/aural communication – the use of the vocal and auditory tract respectively for expressive and receptive communication.

phonology – the sound system of language.

preferred language – this term is used to describe the language a child would most easily acquire and develop to a level most appropriate to their age and development.

prelingual deafness – deafness that has been apparent before a person has begun to develop a language.

postlingual deafness – deafness that has been acquired after the person has partially or fully developed their spoken language.

profound hearing loss – a hearing loss greater than 90 dBHL.

recruitment – the sensation of abnormal loudness growth in relation to input often associated with sensori-neural hearing loss.

semi-circular canals – part of the structure of the inner ear which is concerned with balance.

severe hearing loss – a hearing loss of between 71 dBHL – 95dBHL.

sign language – the visual/gestural language of the deaf community. In the UK this language is British Sign Language; in the USA it is American Sign Language. It is a naturally evolved visual gestural language with its own grammatical structure and lexicon.

sign bilingual – describes an individual who engages with and uses sign language and the language of the hearing community.

transduce – change from one state to another.

Chapter 1

The Ear and How it Works

Anatomy and physiology of the ear

The ear can be divided into three parts. The outer ear, the middle ear and inner ear (Figure 1.1).

The outer ear

The outer ear comprises:

- the pinna or auricle;
- the ear canal or external auditory meatus;
- the ear drum or tympanic membrane.

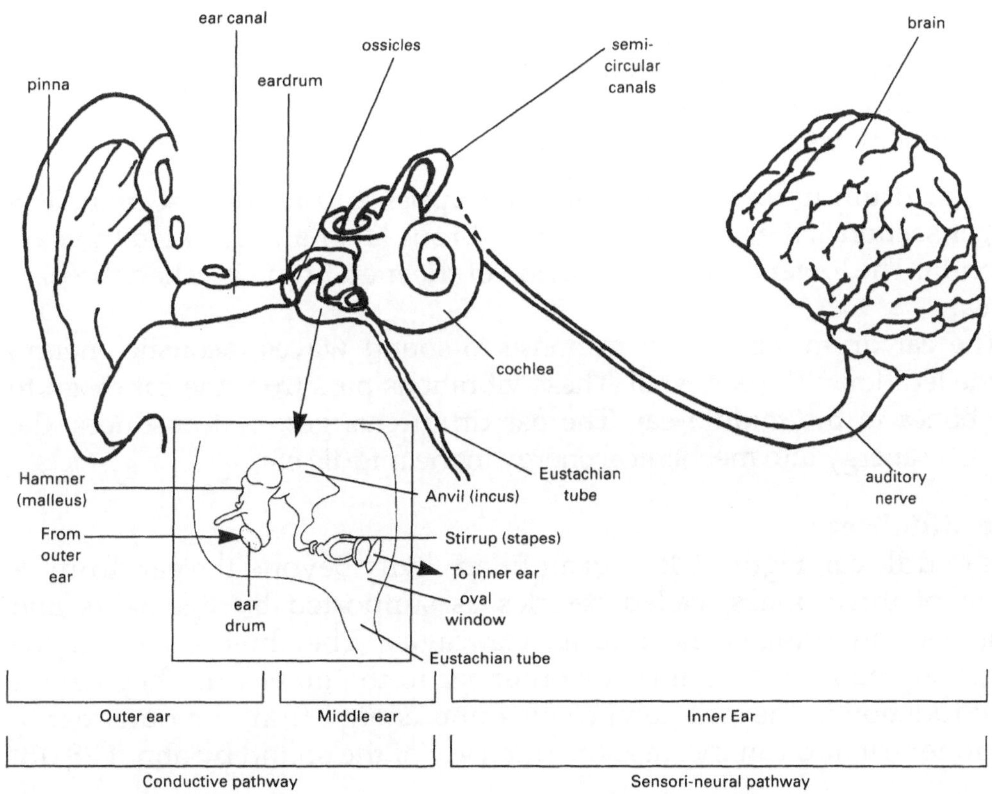

Figure 1.1 The complete hearing system (after Tate 1994)

The pinna or auricle is a structure of pliable cartilage with a tight covering of skin. It is a complex shape designed to collect sound waves, particularly from a forward direction, and funnel them into the ear canal and to the ear drum. The pinna enhances sound reception by about 5dB and assists with the localisation of sound.

The ear canal, or external auditory meatus, is a tube approximately 2.5 cm long which is closed at the inner end by the ear drum or tympanic membrane. The outer third of the ear canal is composed of cartilage, which is continuous from the pinna. This part of the ear canal contains ceruminous glands. These secrete cerumen or wax which helps to protect the ear canal and to moisturise the air in the canal. Wax, which is a mixture of the secretions of sebaceous and sweat glands, mixes with the skin debris which collects in the ear, and migrates naturally outwards, eventually coming out of the ear as a brown moist secretion. Wax is water resistant and inhibits bacterial growth thus protecting the ear from infection. Wax is a natural substance and should not normally be artificially cleaned out of the ear canal.

The inner two thirds of the canal are composed of bone lined with skin, which becomes very thin in the deeper parts of the canal.

The ear drum or tympanic membrane is the membrane found at the end of the canal, separating the outer ear from the middle ear. It is composed of three layers:

- the outer layer is a skin or epithelial layer;
- the middle layer is a fibrous layer;
- the inner layer is a mucosal layer.

The ear drum itself is divided into an upper and a lower section. The upper section is the smaller. It has no fibrous layer and is called the pars flaccida. The lower and larger portion of the membrane is called the pars tensa.

The ear drum vibrates in response to sound waves (acoustic energy) funnelled down the ear canal. These vibrations pass from the ear drum to the bones in the middle ear. The ear drum changes, or transduces, the acoustic energy into mechanical energy in the middle ear.

The middle ear

The middle ear, Figure 1.1, is an air filled cavity beyond the ear drum. A chain of three bones, called ossicles, is supported by ligaments and muscles and bridges the middle ear cavity. The three bones in the ossicular chain serve to link the outer ear to the inner ear. They have a vital function in the transference of sound energy from the outer ear to the inner ear and can increase the intensity of the sound by about 28 dB.

The chain consists of the malleus (hammer) which has a handle and a head. The handle is attached to the ear drum and can be seen though the ear drum by means of an otoscope. The head of the malleus is attached to the incus (anvil) by a joint. The anvil makes contact with the head of the stapes (stirrup). The footplate of the stapes is attached to the oval window, which is the entrance to the inner ear.

Sound passes most effectively through the middle ear when the air pressure in the middle ear is equal to the atmospheric pressure. This pressure equalisation is maintained by the Eustachian tube.

The Eustachian tube is about 3.5 cm long and runs in an inward and downward direction, from the middle ear, opening into the nasopharynx or throat. The function of the Eustachian tube is to balance the air pressure in the middle ear and also to drain the middle ear of any gathering fluid or mucus.

The middle ear also serves to protect the delicate inner ear structures from any potentially damaging noises. In response to loud sounds, especially low frequency (see Chapter 2), the middle ear muscles contract, causing the ossicular chain to stiffen and so transfer sound less effectively.

The middle ear ends at the oval and round windows, which separate the middle ear from the inner ear. These windows are membrane-covered holes in the bony wall of the cochlea.

The inner ear

The inner ear consists of all those parts of the auditory system beyond the middle ear. Sound waves pass through the oval window to the cochlea where they are converted into electrical signals, which travel along the nerve or neural pathways to the auditory centre of brain. The inner ear is concerned with both hearing and with balance. The cochlea is concerned with hearing while the three semi-circular canals are concerned with balance and are part of the vestibular system. The cochlea and the semi-circular canals make up a fluid filled cavity, which is set in the petrous portion of the skull.

The cochlea

The cochlea looks rather like a snail shell, has two and a half coils and is about the size of a pea. A cross-section of the cochlea (see Figure 1.2), allows us to see that the cochlea has three fluid-filled 'galleries'. These are:

- the scala media,
- the scala vestibuli and
- the scala tympani.

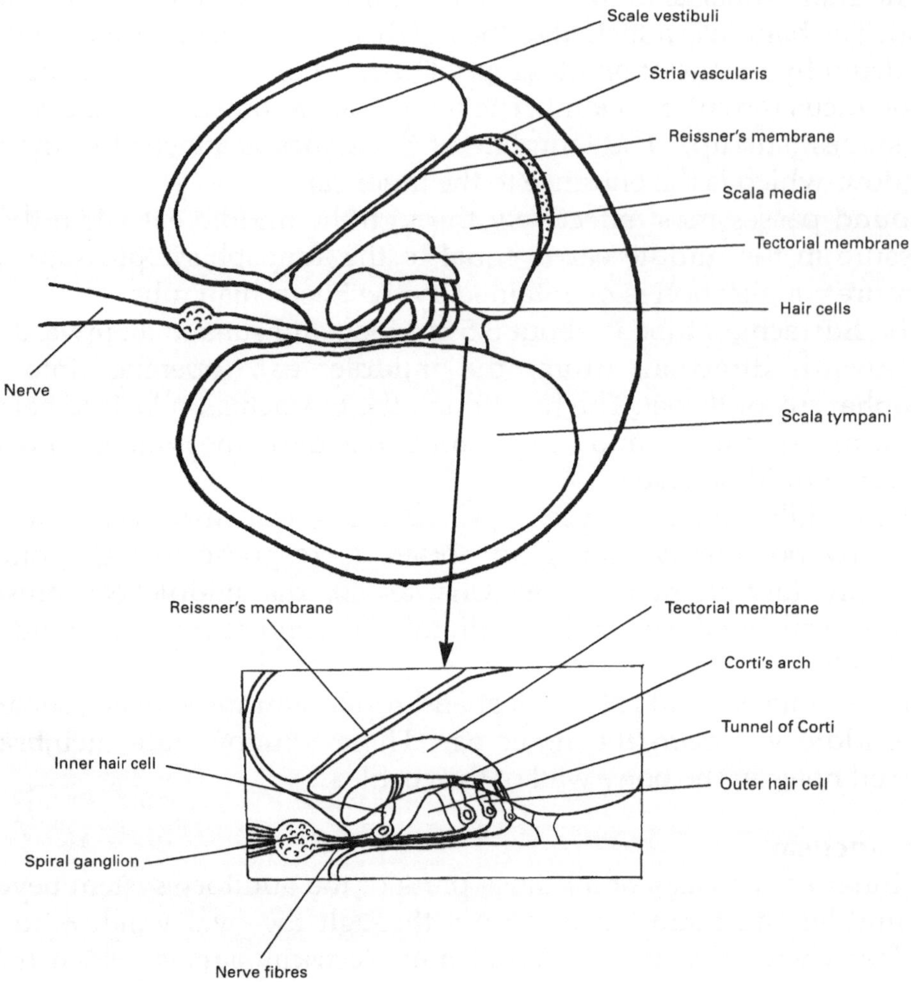

Figure 1.2 Cross-section of the cochlea (after Tate 1994)

The Organ of Corti lies in the central gallery of the cochlea. It consists of rows of hair cells served by nerve fibres. The hair cells are responsible for the transduction of mechanical vibrations received from the middle ear, into electrical impulses. The sound waves travel along the basilar membrane and 'deform' it. Because of the movement, nerve impulses are sent along the nerve fibres. The nerve fibres join to form the auditory nerve, which is part of the eighth cranial nerve. The cochlea is the site where sounds are first analysed into their component frequencies. Different parts of the basilar membrane are sensitive to different frequencies of the sound spectrum (like a piano keyboard). The base of the cochlea is sensitive to high frequency sound waves and the apex of the cochlea is sensitive to low frequency sound waves. All sound waves must travel across the base of the cochlea and maximum 'wear and tear' occurs in this area. Therefore high frequency hearing losses are the most common.

The auditory nerve and brain

The auditory nerve carries the signal to the hearing centres of the brain. The brain interprets frequency according to the part of the cochlea from which the nerve impulses are sent and the intensity according to the number of nerve impulses received.

The area of the brain that is primarily involved in decoding sensory information is the cerebral cortex. Signals from each ear are sent to both left and right hemispheres of the brain but most information is projected to the opposite side of the body. Thus neurons from the left cochlea project predominantly to the right cortex and vice versa. At a functional level, the cortical auditory regions in the left and right hemispheres have different specialisations. The left hemisphere is specialised for language processing (Binder *et al.* 1996) and the right hemisphere for processing music (Penhune *et al.* 1999).

Aetiology: types and causes of deafness

Types of deafness

Audiologically the ear can be divided into conductive and sensori-neural pathways in relation to the transmission of sound energy. The type of deafness is largely related to the place in the hearing system where the cause of deafness is situated.

- *Conductive hearing loss* is deafness resulting from any malfunction or abnormality which prevents or reduces the conduction of sound waves through the outer or middle ear to the oval window of the inner ear.
- *Sensori-neural hearing loss* or 'nerve' deafness is hearing loss that occurs in the inner ear, i.e. the cochlea, the auditory nerve, the auditory pathway or the hearing centres of the brain. This prevents, reduces and distorts the sounds reaching the auditory cortex.
- Mixed hearing loss describes the presence of sensori-neural deafness with some conductive deafness in addition.
- Unilateral or monaural hearing loss is deafness that is apparent in one ear only. It may be conductive or sensori-neural or mixed. The child can hear well in one ear but may have difficulties in noisy surroundings and with locating the direction of sound (see later in this chapter).

Causes of deafness

Most causes of deafness in children fall into three categories:

- hereditary (congenital);
- peri-natal (that which occurs around the birth);
- acquired (occurring during a child's lifetime).

These can affect the conductive pathway, the sensori-neural pathway, or both.

Conductive hearing loss

Causes of conductive hearing loss

Hereditary conductive hearing loss is largely caused by:

- Anatomical abnormalities – these arise in the womb as the ear is developing and can include an absence of the outer ear, atresia (occlusion or closure of the ear canal) and the absence of ossicles.

Peri-natal conductive hearing loss is largely caused by:

- Fluid and debris in the ear canal, which is usually treatable.

Acquired conductive hearing loss is largely caused by:

- Otitis media or inflammation of the middle ear. This is one of the most common disorders in children. The most usual cause is the loss of eustachian tube function, through upper respiratory tract infections (throat and nose infections) impairing the function of the middle ear. This condition, also called glue ear, is discussed further in the following section.
- Foreign bodies – children sometimes push small items, for example beads, into their ears. If these block the ear canal, they will cause some degree of deafness.
- Otitis externa or inflammation of the outer ear. If the ear canal swells or if there is discharge, this may also cause hearing loss. The whole canal can be affected or a localised area. In either case the ear canal is very tender.
- Impacted wax. Wax may accumulate and turn brown and hard in the ear canal . It will cause hearing loss if it blocks the ear canal. This deafness may be accompanied by a 'buzzing' tinnitus.
- Otosclerosis is a condition in which the movement of the stapes is restricted by an abnormal growth of bone in the ossicular chain. (Otosclerosis is a hereditary condition which is not present at birth but which develops later in life).
- Stenosis is a closure or narrowing of the ear canal. (Atresia is similar but present at birth).

Glue ear (Otitis Media)

The most common cause of conductive hearing loss is otitis media, commonly known as 'glue ear'. This is a prevalent condition in children under eight years old. About 15–20 per cent of children in the two to five year age range will have 'glue ear' at any one time. Glue ear gives rise to fluctuating hearing loss, which is largely a passing condition but it is important to realise that when it is present it can significantly affect children's hearing at a crucial time in their linguistic development.

Otitis media occurs when the Eustachian tube is unable to keep the middle ear ventilated, often due to ear or throat infections. Fluid in the middle ear is then also unable to drain away. This problem is most common in young children because the Eustachian tube is narrow and situated horizontally, which impedes ventilation and drainage. As children mature, the Eustachian tube widens and becomes angled downwards towards the throat thus facilitating the drainage process (see Figure 1.3).

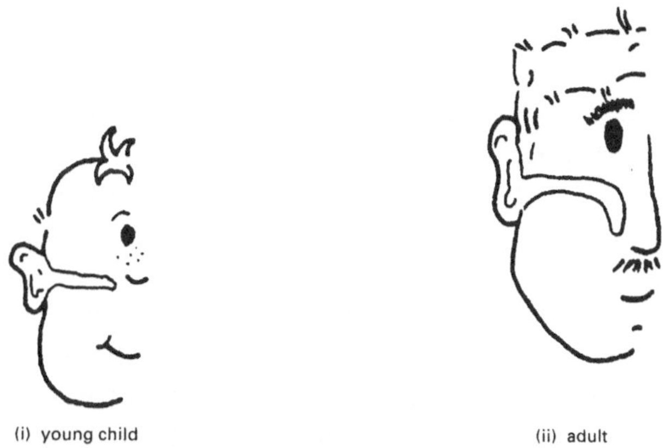

Figure 1.3 The Eustachian tube in child and adult

During ear and throat infections the oxygen in the air in the middle ear is gradually used up and this creates negative pressure (a vacuum) in the middle ear. The ear cannot allow this to happen and to compensate, a watery fluid leaks from the walls of the middle ear, preventing a vacuum from forming. Although at first the fluid is thin and watery, as time passes, it can become thicker and 'glue-like'. Hence the term 'glue ear'. In the medical profession it is also called otitis media with effusion, secretory otitis media, and serous otitis media. These terms are descriptive of the condition along a continuum from the early accumulation of the fluid to the development of glue ear. As the fluid accumulates, it impedes the function of the ossicular chain in the middle ear to transmit sound energy in the form of vibrations. This causes a dullness of hearing, or some degree of deafness, particularly in the low frequencies. The fluid should drain away via the Eustachian tube when the infection is resolved and the tube is no longer blocked. However, if the fluid has reached glue-like thickness the secretion may not be able to drain away even when the infection is resolved. Glue ear may therefore become a long-standing condition. There are implications for children who have frequent bouts of otitis media and glue ear including:

- levels of deafness;
- auditory processing difficulties;
- lower educational attainments;
- restricted language development.

Children with fluid in the ear frequently have hearing loss that fluctuates from day to day and even between the two ears. They have problems associated with the deafness, but also have particular problems due to its fluctuating nature. Fluctuating hearing loss may affect children's ability to localise sound, thus making it difficult for them to identify the person speaking and so they may miss parts of the spoken message. As words may not sound the same from one time to the next, the child's ability to process sound and subsequently develop language may also be impaired. This in turn may affect their educational progress.

An inability to follow conversations easily can lead to issues of behaviour management both at home and in the classroom. Poor acoustic conditions compound the problems for children with glue ear.

Fluid in the middle ear is commonly diagnosed using tympanometry (see Chapter 3). Treatment includes the use of antibiotics and antihistamines for the infection. When the problem is long standing, surgery is often undertaken to insert grommets (see Figure 1.4). This minor operation involves making a small hole in the ear drum through which the fluid is removed. The hole is then kept open for a period of time by inserting a ventilation tube (grommet). There are several types of grommet including a T tube grommet commonly used for long term ventilation of the middle ear. The hole in the eardrum gradually heals and the grommet then naturally comes out via the ear canal.

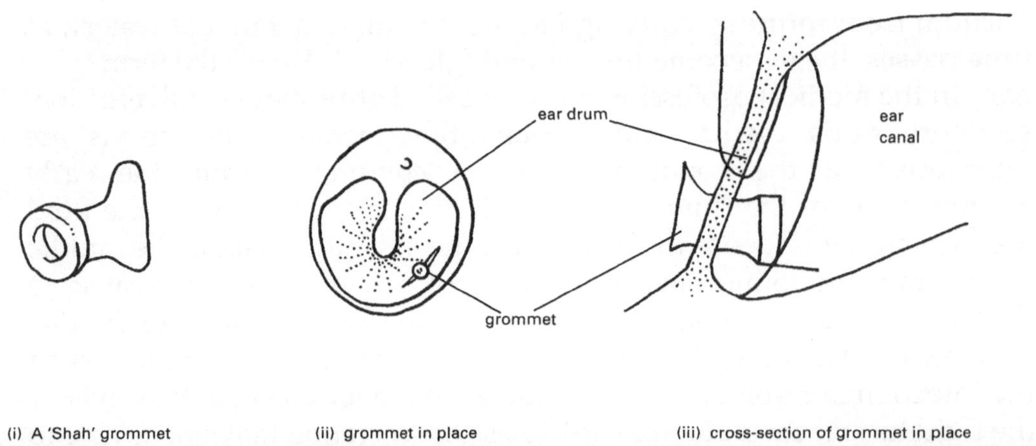

Figure 1.4 Grommets (after Tate 1994 and Ballantyne 1993)

Effects of conductive hearing loss on sound perception
In conductive hearing loss, sound is prevented, to a greater or lesser degree, from reaching the inner ear. All sounds are available to the inner ear but the loudness (intensity) will be reduced or not perceived at all. Although with a conductive hearing loss the sounds reaching the inner ear may be reduced in intensity, they are not distorted. Generally conductive deafness can be addressed medically and at least responds well to the use of hearing aids.

Sensori-neural or nerve hearing loss

Causes of sensori-neural hearing loss
The most common cause of sensori-neural hearing loss is maturity (age-related hearing loss is called 'presbyacusis'). The majority of adults over the age of 50 years will begin to experience some loss of hearing acuity, generally in the high frequency range of hearing. Most sensori-neural hearing loss both in adults and children primarily affects the high frequencies of the sound spectrum. Other causes of sensori-neural hearing loss in children include:

Congenital causes:

- Genetic: Inherited deafness is related to the chromosomatic makeup of the parents. Chromosomes determine all our physical functions including hearing. There are dominant (or active) and recessive (or weaker) chromosomes. The dominant one governs the hearing status of the child. It is the match of chromosomes between parents that affects the hearing status of the child and it is possible for one parent to have a dominant chromosome which is a carrier of sensori-neural hearing loss even though they themselves are hearing.
- Infection in expectant mothers, e.g. maternal rubella, cytomegalovirus (CMV) and syphilis, can cause sensori-neural hearing loss and other developmental problems in babies. (Deafness through maternal rubella has been largely addressed by early inoculation). The effect upon the developing embryo depends to a great extent upon the stage of the pregnancy. Infection in early pregnancy is the most likely cause of damage to the unborn child.

Peri-natal causes (around birth):

- prematurity – some sensori-neural hearing loss is known to occur in cases of severe prematurity, although improved medical intervention can address many of the issues arising.
- anoxia – lack of oxygen to the baby immediately after birth is thought

to be linked to sensori-neural hearing loss, although identification of 'at risk' babies has ameliorated this problem to a large extent.

- jaundice – is related to high levels of bilirubin in the blood which result in jaundice. This damages the nerve of hearing at the brain stem.
- rhesus incompatibility – this is related to the blood grouping which can be either rhesus positive or negative. If a mother with a positive rhesus factor is carrying a baby with a negative rhesus factor then anti-bodies form in the blood of the mother and can be passed onto the baby with possible harmful effects to the baby, and their hearing mechanism. This situation is well documented and largely addressed by medical intervention.

Acquired causes (post-natal):

- bacterial and viral infections, e.g. mumps, measles and meningitis, which may affect one or both ears. These are the most common causes of unilateral hearing loss;
- head injuries;
- ototoxic drugs e.g. streptomycin, quinine etc.
- over-exposure to loud noise;
- tumours on the acoustic nerve.

Effects of sensori-neural hearing loss on sound perception

Sensori-neural hearing loss is a result of damage to the inner ear and is generally permanent. It is likely to be the result of local damage to a particular site in the cochlea or group of nerve fibres. Therefore this form of deafness can produce both distortions in sound perception, where specific frequencies of sound may be affected, and also reduced responses to sound. An example of this is in high tone hearing loss where response to high frequency tones is seriously affected, while that for low tones may be near to normal. This causes a distortion in the auditory information arriving at the auditory cortex.

Implications of unilateral hearing loss

Children with unilateral hearing loss are often considered by the general public as having 'normal hearing', because they tend to manage well in most situations. Unilaterally deaf children may produce good free-field speech test results in quiet conditions, have no speech production problems, use the telephone, hear the television and have no noticeable difficulty in understanding. Clearly the degree of deafness is a factor in the potential difficulties caused by unilateral hearing loss, but teachers should not underestimate those difficulties. These include:

- hearing sounds on the affected side.
- localising sound (identifying the direction of the sound source).
- listening to and understanding speech in the presence of background noise.

Visual clues are important to the unilaterally deaf child to supplement auditory information and seating should allow a clear view of any visual supplement. Additional support should be implemented early if there is evidence of significant educational need. Listening through an FM radio system (individual or sound field, depending on the degree of hearing loss) can be very successful (see Chapter 6). Teachers should also be sensitive to the need to protect the child's good ear from potential damage, for example from loud noise.

Tinnitus

Tinnitus is the subjective sensation of noise, without any external cause. It may appear in the ears or in the head and common descriptions include whistles, hissing, throbbing and buzzing. It can be intermittent or continuous and is very common in conjunction with deafness. Deaf children may have tinnitus but in most cases it is not a particular problem and many who have it do not realise that it is not the norm.

Non-organic hearing loss

There are children who appear to be deaf while in fact they do not have a significant hearing loss, or where their deafness is not as severe as it seems. Non-organic hearing loss refers to the condition in which there is no apparent bodily (organic) cause for the hearing problem. Non-organic hearing loss in adults is usually false (malingering) for compensation purposes. In children non-organic hearing loss should always be seen as a symptom of an underlying problem and psychological help is often needed. Children with non-organic hearing loss usually give signs of inconsistency such as exaggerated reliance on lip-reading or good speech discrimination despite test results indicating severe deafness.

Summary

- The ear is divided into the outer, middle and inner ear and the anatomy and physiology of the ear is described.
- Conductive hearing loss occurs in either the outer or the middle ear and results in the reduction of sound level but does not distort the sound. It is usually medically treatable and also responds well to the use of hearing aids.

- Sensori-neural hearing loss occurs in the inner ear. Sounds are reduced in intensity and are also distorted. Sensori-neural deafness is rarely reversible and although hearing aids help, it is more difficult to aid this type of loss efficiently.

Further reading

Maltby, M. (2001) Chapter 2 'Anatomy and physiology of the ear' and Chapter 3 'Medical aspects of hearing loss', in *Principles of Hearing Aid Audiology*, 2nd edn. London: Whurr Publishers.

Chapter 2

The Physics of Hearing

An introduction to sound

Sound requires a source, a medium through which to travel, and a detector. The source of sound is a vibrating body, e.g. a drum, a tuning fork or vocal cords, and the sound generated is transmitted through a medium or substance which is generally air but may be any elastic medium: gas, liquid or solid. The detector is usually a listener but could be any sound measuring device, such as a sound level meter.

In air, the sound source sets the air particles into vibration in the same back and forth motion as the vibrating source. The medium, through which the vibrations travel, is not itself transferred to the detector. The sound energy is passed across the medium in a series of pressure variations called compressions and rarefactions. In compression, the air particles move closer together and in rarefaction they move further apart. Each compression and rarefaction constitutes one cycle of a sound wave.

The speed of sound varies with the medium through which it is travelling. The denser the medium, the faster sound travels. Sounds become weaker with increasing distance from the source.

The simplest sound wave form is a pure tone (see Figure 2.1). All sounds, no matter how complex, are made up of a combination of individual pure tones. Study of basic acoustics considers the nature of sound at the level of the pure tone. The major characteristics of a pure tone are the:

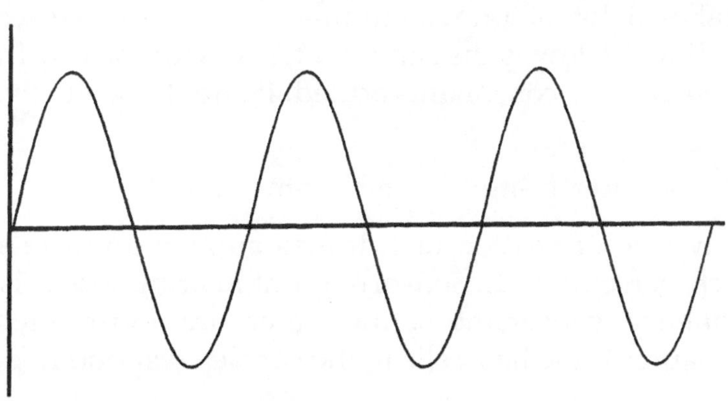

Figure 2.1 A sound wave consisting of one pure tone

- frequency (pitch);
- intensity (loudness);
- phase.

Frequency (pitch)

Frequency is subjectively experienced as pitch. Frequency (pitch) is measured in hertz (Hz). The term hertz is used to describe the number of cycles which occur per second in the sound wave. For example a tone of 250 Hz would complete 250 cycles per second, a 4,000 Hz tone would complete 4,000 cycles per second. Middle C on the piano is about 260 Hz.

The young, healthy human ear is capable of hearing sounds from approximately 20 Hz (very low sounds) to 20,000 Hz (very high sounds) but the frequencies of speech fall usually between 125 Hz and 8,000 Hz, and the most important speech frequencies fall between 250 Hz and 4000Hz.

Speech frequencies vary across the speech range from the low frequency vowel sounds e.g. 'u' or 'o' and nasal sounds e.g. 'n' or 'm' to the higher frequency consonant sounds e.g. 'f','s','sh','th'.

Low frequency sounds		**Middle frequency sounds**		**High frequency sounds**	
a	as in cat	ay	as in day	s	as in sink
oo	as in mood	ee	as in weed	sh	as in ship
ow	as in how	d	as in do	f	as in fence
or	as in bored	m	as in mouse	th	as in think

Table 2.1 Examples of speech sounds within each frequency range

In general terms, the vowels (lower frequency sounds of speech) contribute power to speech, and also information about rhythm and intonation. The consonants (higher frequency sounds) contribute to the intelligibility of speech and give the meaning.

For example, look at the following sentence:

I a- -oi-- -o -e- -o-e --ee--

This is a simple sentence with all the high frequency consonant sounds removed. It takes a lot of understanding (unless you are especially skilled at decoding). Below is the same sentence with the low frequency vowels removed and the consonants added. It should be much easier to understand:

- -m g--ng t- g-t s-m- sw--ts

This is certainly true of written text. It also appears to have a similar effect on speech perception. In sensori-neural hearing loss it is usually the high frequency consonant sounds that are most affected. As described in Chapter 1, the hair cells in the cochlea respond to particular frequencies and those nearest the oval window, which relay high frequency sounds, are most vulnerable to damage. They are often badly distorted and may be missing totally in severe cases.

Severe sensori-neural deafness presents problems of both reduced loudness and distortion of speech sounds, particularly for young deaf children developing spoken language.

Intensity (loudness)

Intensity is subjectively experienced as loudness. The sound pressure level (SPL) or intensity is a measure of how much pressure is generated by the sound source. The greater the deviation of the compression and rarefaction of the wave, the higher the pressure and therefore the more intense the sound.

Hearing is non-linear with regard to sound pressure or intensity. When a sound has doubled in energy, it does not appear to be double in loudness. A sound has to increase tenfold in sound energy to appear twice as loud to the listener. This is a logarithmic response.

relative intensity	related sound
1	just audible
1000	whisper
1000 000	normal speech
1000 000 000	loud shout
1000 000 000 000	discomfort level

Table 2.2 The range of intensities the human ear can handle

A scale of intensity ranging from 1 to 1 000 000 000 000 is very clumsy to use and would be misleading. By taking the logarithm of the intensities, the very large intensity ratios become more manageable as well as more realistic. This logarithmic unit is called the bel after Alexander Graham Bell. The bel has been divided into tenths (decibels) and is abbreviated to dB.

It is accepted practice to measure the intensity of any particular sound in decibels (dB). The decibel scales express the ratio between two numbers. To be meaningful, a ratio must have a reference level. It may help to remember that if you say one thing is stronger than something else, you need to say *what* it is stronger than; this is its reference level. Thus, for example, 20dBHL is 20dB more intense than the quietest sound the normally hearing ear can detect, which is established as 0 dBHL. This is its reference level.

There are a number of dB scales and the teacher is likely to come across the dBHL, dBSPL and dBA scales. These are explained below.

The dBHL scale

The level at which sound is just perceived is called threshold. Hearing thresholds are measured using the dBHL (decibel hearing level) scale. When using the dBHL scale, the level of sound is described by comparison to average normal hearing. The normal ear is most sensitive to sounds in the mid-frequency region. This is the frequency region most important for understanding speech. The ear, however, is not equally sensitive to all sounds across the audible frequency range. Very high frequency and very low frequency sounds, for example, have to be more intense to be heard. The actual sound pressure levels for 0dBHL (threshold) vary at each frequency and are given in the British Standards (BS 2497: Part 5: 1988).

The 'average' normally hearing person has a threshold of 0dBHL. Sounds begin to be uncomfortably loud at about 120dBHL and intolerably painful at about 140dBHL. A graph of hearing threshold is known as the audiogram. When hearing is tested, the results are usually plotted on an audiogram. The dBHL scale is used whenever hearing is tested under headphones.

The dB(A) scale

The response of the human ear in the sound field (e.g. in a room) is slightly different to the response when listening through headphones. Like the dBHL scale, the dB(A) scale has normal hearing threshold as its reference level, but it is normal hearing threshold not wearing headphones. The dBHL scale is based on hearing through each ear separately, whereas the dB(A) scale is based on binaural hearing. The dB(A) scale provides values that are about 4dB greater than the dBHL scale. This is partly because hearing is improved when both ears are used together.

The A-weighted scale was designed for use at low (quiet) levels of sound but is now used almost exclusively in noise measurement. Table 2.3 gives an indication of the approximate intensity levels of some everyday sounds.

Sound Intensity in Decibels (dBA)	
0 dB	the quietest sound the healthy ear can detect (pin drop)
20 dB	a whisper at 1 meter
40 dB	a quiet conversation
60 dB	normal conversation
80 dB	a shout
100 dB	a road drill
120 dB	an aircraft taking off
140 dB	normal threshold of pain (jet take off at 25m.)

Table 2.3 Approximate intensities of everyday sounds

The dBSPL scale

The dBSPL (sound pressure level) scale relates to variations in sound pressure. It takes no account of the way human hearing varies across the frequency range, for example at mid frequencies we can hear less intense sound pressures than at very low or very high frequencies.

The international unit of pressure is the Pascal (Pa). The dBSPL scale has 0.00002 Pa as its reference pressure (0dBSPL). This is the smallest amount of sound pressure at 1kHz, which is audible to the average normally hearing person. 0dBSPL at each frequency is 0.00002 Pa, regardless of whether or not it would be audible to the human ear. At 1kHz, the dBSPL scale is fairly similar to the dBHL scale but, at very high and very low frequencies, dBSPL measurements are very different to those recorded in dBHL.

The dBSPL scale is used in hearing aid testing. Teachers need to understand that hearing aid data therefore cannot be related directly to the pure tone audiogram. Ideally, the teacher should compare the child's results using the same test (for example free field audiograms or speech tests). Alternatively, an estimate of benefit can be obtained by looking at the gain or amplification provided by the aid (see Chapter 9) and adding this to the child's unaided levels.

Phase and phase cancellation.

As we have seen, a sound wave consists of a series of compressions (regions of increased pressure) and rarefactions (regions of decreased pressure). The phase of the wave simply refers to the stage in its progression, for example, let us consider one cycle of a pure tone wave-form, in Figure 2.2.

If we consider two such wave-forms, they are said to be exactly in phase when corresponding points of the wave-forms coincide at exactly the same point in time, as shown in Figure 2.3.

If these two waves arrived together at the listener's ear in phase, then they would combine constructively to form a larger amplitude wave-form of the same frequency, ie. perceived as louder than its constituents.

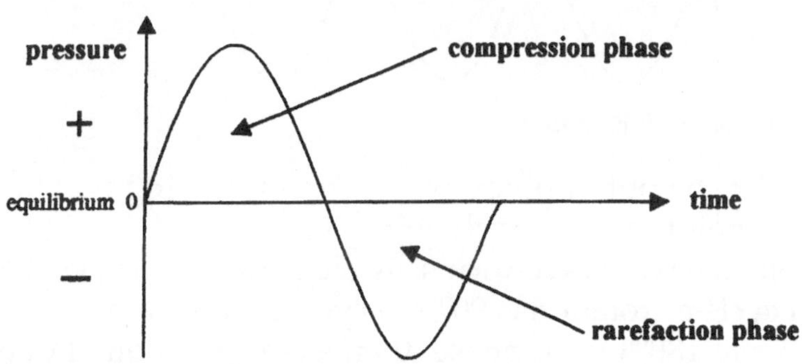

Figure 2.2 Phases of a pure tone

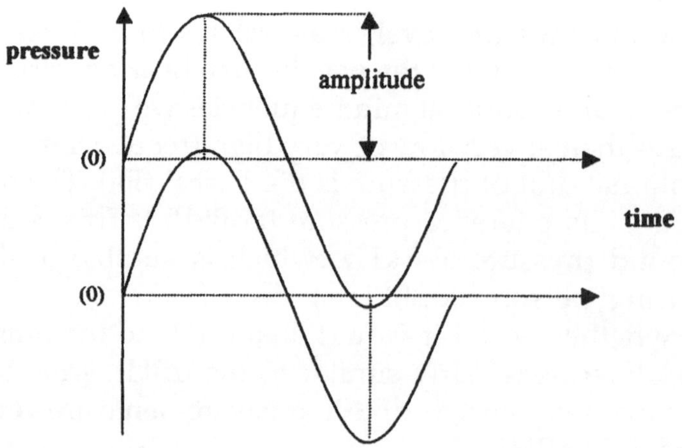

Figure 2.3 Pure tones in phase

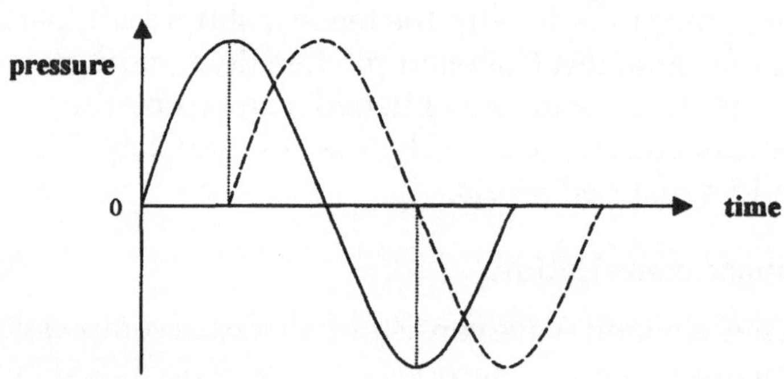

Figure 2.4 Pure tones out of phase

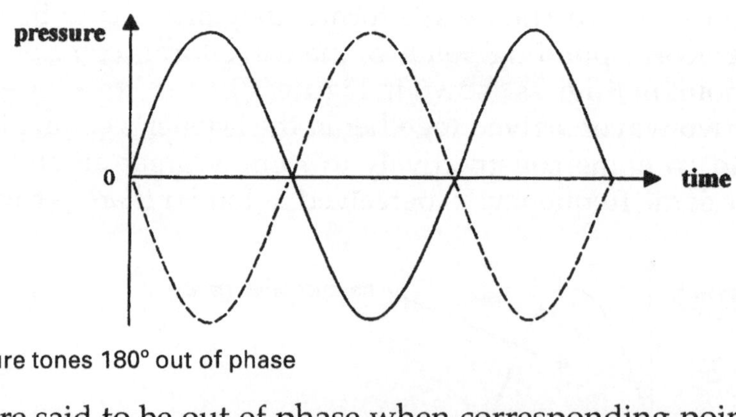

Figure 2.5 Pure tones 180° out of phase

Waves are said to be out of phase when corresponding points do not occur at the same point in time, as shown in Figure 2.4.

In this example, the two wave-forms are a quarter of a cycle or 90° out of phase (¼ of a cycle or rotation is 90°, ½ a cycle is 180° etc.).

If the waves were 180° out of phase, then a compression of one wave would coincide exactly with a rarefaction of the other (see Figure 2.5).

If these two waves combined, they would do so *destructively* and would cancel each other out and the resultant wave-form would be, in this extreme case, a flat line, ie. no sound would be perceived.

This type of destructive interference is termed phase cancellation. This has several implications for testing and hearing aid fitting, for example, 'dead spots' would occur in free field testing if pure tones were used, and many digital hearing aids use phase cancellation to reduce acoustic feedback (whistling).

Hearing threshold

The point at which pure tones are just audible is called the threshold of hearing. This is determined using pure tone audiometry (see Chapter 3). The threshold of hearing is specific to the individual. The standard threshold of hearing (0dBHL) is established on the basis of a statistical average obtained by testing many otologically normal young people. The hearing area lies between the threshold of hearing and the threshold of discomfort. For the average normally hearing person this lies between 0dBHL and approximately 120dBHL, giving a 'dynamic range' of 120dB (120–0).

Audiograms

When a hearing test is carried out, the hearing threshold is measured over a range of frequencies. These are then plotted on an audiogram.

The vertical axis on the audiogram indicates the intensity of sound. The quietest sound that normally hearing children can perceive will be in the region of –10 to +10 dBHL. Normal hearing in adults is generally defined as 20 dBHL or better, but *any* degree of hearing loss may disadvantage a school child.

The horizontal axis indicates the frequency of sound. Normally hearing people will detect all sounds across the frequency range tested. The range normally tested in audiometry, and presented on audiograms, is from 250Hz to 8kHz. The frequency range most important to the understanding of speech is between about 250Hz and 4kHz.

The hearing levels of each ear may be plotted on the same or separate audiograms. Standard symbols are used to avoid confusion:

- the right ear is represented by **O** (often coloured red)
- the left ear is represented by **X** (often coloured blue).

The points plotted are joined to give a graphic representation of the hearing loss for each ear, as shown in Figure 2.6.

Speech perception

The component sounds of speech can be plotted according to their individual frequency and intensity value.

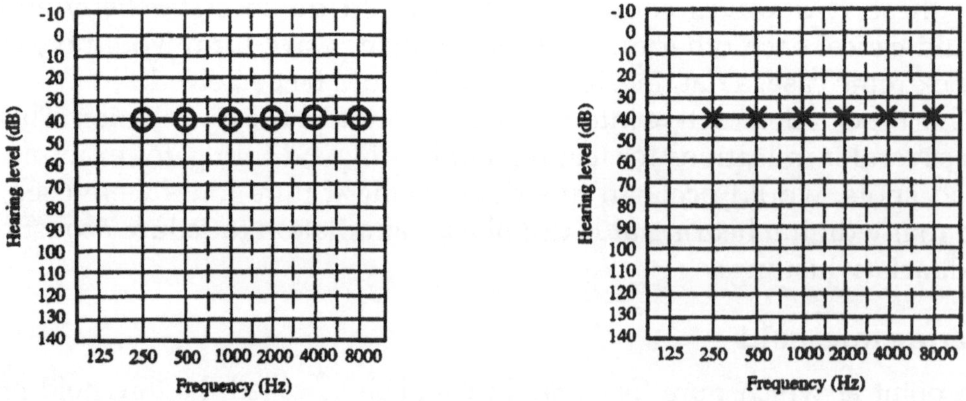

Key: Right Left
Air conduction, masked if necessary ○ ×

Figure 2.6 An audiogram showing a 40dB hearing loss (diagram courtesy of A&M Hearing Ltd)

There is a wide variation in the intensity of the individual components of running speech. The loudest sounds are vowels and the quietest sounds are consonants. The quietest sounds in speech are approximately 30dB less intense than the loudest sounds. This variation in intensity remains the same regardless of the overall power of the speech sound. In other words, whether speech is quiet or loud, the variation in intensity between the individual sounds remains the same.

The outlined part within the audiogram in Figure 2.7 indicates the average range of speech energy in dBHL. This area is sometimes called the 'speech banana'. The softest speech sounds will appear near the upper boundary of the speech area and the loudest sounds will fall near the lower boundary. It can also be seen that speech sounds fall mainly into the frequency range from 400 Hz to 6,000Hz (6kHz).

When hearing thresholds fall below the speech area, some or all components of speech will be reduced in intensity or lost altogether. By considering audiograms that represent different types and degrees of deafness, in relation to the 'speech banana', it becomes possible to understand how speech perception may be affected.

Description of hearing level

Whenever the hearing level is worse than normal, there is said to be a hearing loss. The layman tends to refer to all levels of hearing loss as 'deafness'. Audiologists tend to refer to levels of hearing loss rather than deafness, at least for less severe levels. The terminology used is not 'right or wrong', but is sometimes seen as being 'politically correct'.

Average normal hearing will appear as a flat line across the top of the audiogram. However, degrees of hearing loss are rarely simple. When

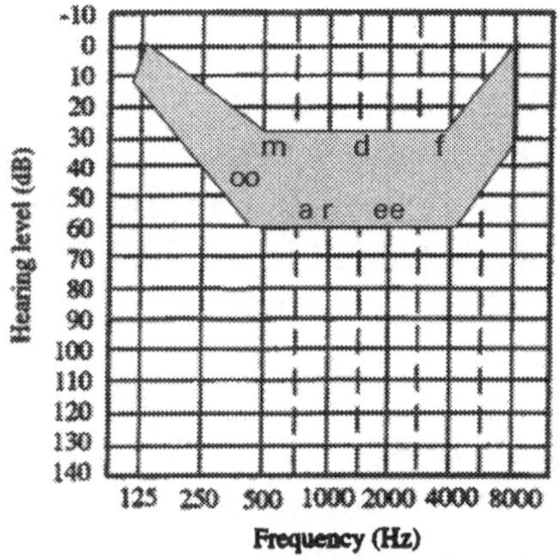

Figure 2.7 An audiogram showing the area in which conversational speech falls, 'the speech banana', and some speech sounds (diagram courtesy of A&M Hearing Ltd)

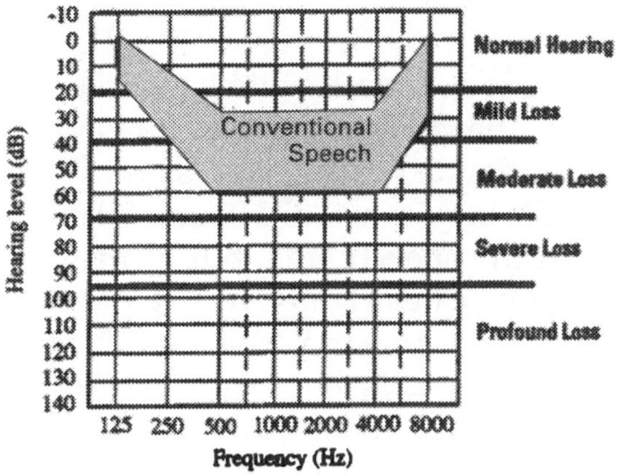

Figure 2.8 An audiogram showing the various hearing levels and degrees of hearing loss (diagram courtesy of A&M Hearing Ltd)

the hearing loss is averaged, it will fall into a particular category of degree of loss, for example moderate. When it is viewed on the audiogram, however, the loss may not appear flat and may span more than one category, for example moderate to severe.

Hearing loss may therefore be described according to the slope of the loss as well as the degree. In addition, the type of hearing loss, which may be sensori-neural, conductive or mixed, will affect how the child hears.

Degrees of hearing level

The audiogram in Figure 2.8 shows different degrees of hearing level. The outline of the speech 'banana' is included on the audiogram to provide an indication of how much of the speech signal is likely to be lost when the hearing is not aided.

Normal hearing is generally accepted as falling within the band –10dBHL to 20dBHL, and should therefore appear as a fairly flat line across the top of the audiogram form. This line or 'curve' shows the threshold (this is the level at which sounds can just be detected) of normal hearing. Both ears should appear broadly similar. Comfortable conversational levels are about 30–40 dB louder than the threshold.

The average hearing level is usually calculated, for the better ear, from the average of the most important frequencies for hearing speech. These are generally taken to be the five frequencies: 250Hz, 500Hz, 1kHz, 2kHz and 4kHz. Any hearing loss may then be categorised as: normal, mild, moderate, severe or profound. For accurate calculations see Appendix 1 on audiological descriptors.

A mild hearing loss is one in which the average hearing loss (in the better ear) falls between 20dBHL and 40 dBHL. With this degree of hearing loss, speech will be heard but it will be quieter than usual. Only sounds that are quieter than threshold levels will not be heard at all.

A moderate hearing loss is one in which the average loss (in the better ear) falls between 41dBHL and 70 dBHL. This degree of loss falls largely within the speech area, but at its lower level, and normal speech will therefore be heard only very faintly.

A severe hearing loss is one in which the average loss (in the better ear) falls between 71dBHL and 95 dBHL. This degree of hearing loss falls mainly or entirely outside the speech area. With this degree of loss, general conversation will not be heard and loud sounds will be heard only as quiet sounds.

A profound hearing loss is one in which the average loss (in the better ear) falls below 95 dBHL. With this degree of loss, nothing of speech will be heard and even with hearing aids speech will appear distorted. Communication will rely very heavily on visual skills.

Descriptors of hearing loss

The hearing loss is often described by its shape on the audiogram, as well as by the degree of loss. Commonly used descriptors include: flat, sloping, ski-slope and left-hand corner.

A flat loss is one in which the hearing level does not vary much across the frequency range. A sloping loss is one in which the hearing level falls off across the frequency range. A sloping loss may be gradual or it may fall off steeply. A steeply falling loss is often referred to as a 'ski-slope'. Sloping losses are usually worst in the high frequency region; this is the most common shape of all hearing losses. When a hearing loss is worst in the low frequencies, it may be referred to as a 'reverse slope'.

Where there is very little hearing remaining ('residual hearing'), the audiogram may consist only of a few points near the bottom of the audiogram and in the low frequency region; this configuration is often referred to as a 'left-hand corner' audiogram.

Sloping losses in which the hearing for high frequency sounds is worst are the most common configuration of sensori-neural hearing loss. With this shape of loss, the low frequency sounds tend to be heard well. These sounds are mainly vowel sounds, which give volume and rhythm to speech. The high frequency consonant sounds are reduced or lost. This affects the clarity of speech and makes it difficult to understand. Teachers need to be very aware of the difficulties caused by sloping losses as these can be much greater than they may appear at first sight.

Where the loss is a 'ski-slope' this problem is magnified as the hearing in the low frequencies may be more or less normal while that in the high frequencies falls off rapidly, often falling into the profound category.

Commonly young children with this type of loss begin to talk at the usual time but their expressive speech will sound 'different' as some speech sounds will be missing and they may be unintelligible to the unfamiliar listener. The main problem in the classroom occurs because low frequency vowel sounds of speech are likely to be heard at normal levels making it appear that the child is hearing well. However, even with hearing aids, the high frequency consonant sounds will be heard only partially. This means that speech will be 'heard' in the sense that the child will be aware of speech via the low frequency sounds but what they hear is likely to be very distorted. Understanding is easier in quiet one-to-one situations in which the child can lip read, and where background noise is not reducing the part of the message that can be heard.

A 'left-hand corner' audiogram refers to a profound hearing loss where the child responds to sound only in the low frequency range. No speech will be heard unaided, and even with powerful hearing aids only the rhythm and intonation of the low frequency sounds of speech are perceived.

Summary

Sound energy has three major characteristics:

- frequency;
- intensity;
- phase.

The frequency of sound is measured in kilohertz (kHz) and the intensity of sound is measured in decibels (dB). Pure tones are sounds consisting of only one frequency.

Hearing thresholds are plotted on a graph called an audiogram. This graph gives a clear indication of the lowest level at which pure tones, within the speech frequency range, can be heard by the person being tested. Audiograms need to be interpreted with care; each is individual to the particular child and they show only what the child can hear in terms of pure tones. They should be used by the teacher as a guide to what each individual is likely to perceive with their residual hearing. There are many factors that influence how well children are able to use their residual hearing.

Further reading

Maltby, M. (2001) Chapter 1: 'Acoustics', in *Principles of Hearing Aid Audiology*, 2nd edn. London: Whurr Publishers.

Northern, J.L. and Downs, M.P. (latest edition) Chapter 1: 'What is hearing loss?', in *Hearing in Children*. Baltimore: Williams and Wilkins.

Chapter 3

Assessment of Hearing Loss

Hearing tests

There is a wide range of hearing tests that can be used with adults and children. The usual way of measuring hearing loss in adults and in children over about four years of age is with pure tone audiometry. For children under the age of four, assessment is more informal, using behavioural observations and 'play'. These tests tend to be undertaken in the sound field (also called the 'free field').

Sound field or free field audiometry refers to testing undertaken using a sound stimulus delivered at a distance from the ear, not under headphones. The intensity of the sound signal is measured using a sound level meter.

The choice of hearing tests in young children is largely dependent upon the child's developmental age.

Tests for assessing levels of deafness fall broadly into two categories, screening and diagnostic.

Screening and diagnostic tests

Screening tests, sometimes called 'sweep tests', may be routinely carried out on new-born babies (neonatal screening), babies of 7–9 months and on entry into school. Hearing is tested across a frequency range at a fixed level, often 30–35dB(A) for babies and 25 dBHL for school-aged children. They are pass or fail tests. Any child failing the screening test is normally sent for more stringent diagnostic testing and assessment in a hospital or clinic, under controlled acoustic conditions.

Any concern expressed by parents, at any stage, should always lead to further testing of hearing. In the vast majority of cases, parents suspect a hearing loss before it is clinically diagnosed (Webster 1997).

The screening test for 7–9 month old infants is a 'distraction test' (see later in this chapter). This needs to be carried out by appropriately trained health visitors as it is possible to get false negative results due to, for example, boredom, sleepiness or distress on the part of the infant, or to get false positive results caused by testers or parents.

School screening is a shortened form of pure tone audiometry, which is performed at selected frequencies and at a fixed intensity level. This test is useful in identifying all types of hearing loss including those that are unilateral, since each ear is tested separately. Screening frequently identifies children who have developed otitis media with effusion (OME) or 'glue ear' but children with mild losses, less than the fixed intensity level of the test, will not be identified. If there remains any suspicion that a child's hearing is impaired, the child should be referred for a diagnostic assessment, irrespective of the school screening result.

The aim of diagnostic testing is to establish the precise degree and nature of deafness in order to take appropriate action: medical, acoustical (amplification), educational or any combination of these. Audiometric tests are used in the prescription of appropriate amplification devices. They are also used to aid understanding of the likely implications for the development of speech and language, for learning and classroom organisation.

Behavioural tests

Pure tone audiometry (described in a later section) is the most common form of hearing assessment but is not possible with very young children. There is a range of tests and testing techniques that have been developed for use with infants. This chapter describes these hearing assessments from a developmental perspective.

Most testing of very young children relies on observation of their behaviour in response to exposure to sound, the level of which is carefully monitored under structured conditions. These tests are known as behavioural tests of hearing.

Behavioural observation audiometry (BOA) (0–6 months)

Behavioural observation audiometry may be used with infants under 6 months of age, or developmentally delayed children, who are not yet able to sit and therefore cannot be tested by distraction methods. Behavioural observation audiometry only identifies a response to sound, it does not establish the threshold of hearing. It relies on presenting a sound to stimulate an observable reaction in the child. Various sound stimuli may be employed; these include speech, bands of noise, warble tones and pre-measured sound-making toys. Behaviours, which may be observed in babies when they are awake or asleep, include:

- eye-widening or eye blinking;
- eye shift or head movement towards the source of sound;
- stilling or quieting;
- stirring or arousal (from sleep);
- increased or decreased sucking movements;
- increased movement of the arms, legs or body.

This test depends upon the observer making a judgement about what is or is not a valid response. Ideally, therefore, there should be two observers looking for behavioural changes. The use of video recording is also helpful in reducing the issue of observer subjectivity. Behavioural observation audiometry is of limited clinical usefulness but may alert the audiologist to those children needing further testing, usually using evoked response audiometry (ERA), discussed later in this chapter.

The auropalpebral reflex (APR)

The auropalpebral reflex (APR) or startle reflex is an involuntary eyeblink, sometimes accompanied by a head jerk, in response to a loud sound. It can be readily observed in most normally hearing babies, children and adults in response to the shout of 'baa' close to the ear (with the mouth covered to avoid cues). Usually this is at about 80 dB above threshold. Results from an APR provide useful but limited results. The absence of a startle reflex does not necessarily indicate a hearing problem, nor does the presence of a startle reflex indicate normal hearing. The presence of an APR only tells us that there is some hearing at the level tested.

The distraction test (6–18 months)

In order to carry out this test the child needs to be able to sit up and turn to locate a sound source. The sound is presented at ear level out of the child's line of vision.

Two testers carry out the test in a quiet room. The child is sitting upon their carer's knee, facing forward. One tester is facing the child, offering the required level of distraction to gain the child's attention, without fully engrossing the child. Usually a small toy is used for this. The second tester, who is positioned behind the child as shown in Figure 3.1, presents a sound signal. At the precise moment of presentation of sound, the toy is covered so that the child momentarily loses interest in the toy and will turn towards the sound.

The object of the test is to record the quietest level at which the child responds to a range of sounds that are frequency specific. These are usually:

- human voice (low frequency);
- G chime bar (middle frequency);
- high frequency rattle.

Although this appears to be a simple test, it requires training and experience to be used effectively, as well as close cooperation between the testers. Sounds must be presented during the brief moment of loss of interest when the toy is covered, and both the distance from the child (usually one metre) and dB level at the child's ear must be measured. The testers also observe the child's localisation of sound.

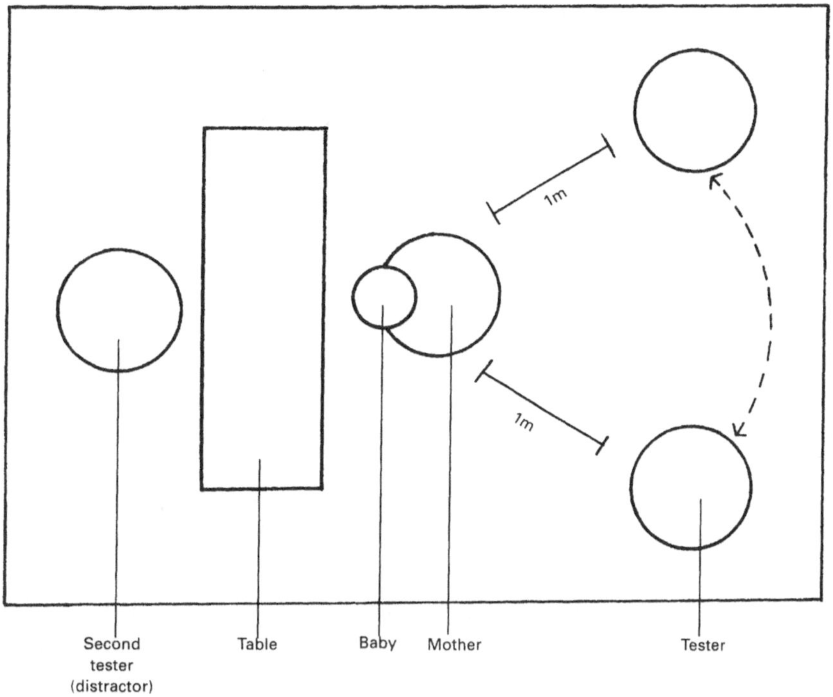

Figure 3.1 The distraction testing set up

Throughout the test, it is important not to give the child any additional cues, or clues, such as:

- coming within the child's peripheral vision;
- casting shadows;
- offering other sensory clues, such as perfume;
- visual communication between the testers.

Visual reinforcement audiometry (VRA) (6–36 months)

An alternative to distraction testing that is sometimes used is VRA. This requires more complex equipment but can be very successful with young children right through to the stage when they are ready for pure tone audiometry. Most commonly in this test, frequency specific tones (usually warble tones or narrow band noise) are delivered at a known frequency, via a loudspeaker. When the child turns in response to the sound, reinforcement is provided, for example, by flashing lights or dancing puppets. Thresholds over the range 500Hz–4 kHz can be reliably obtained, but the results are not left or right specific where the test is delivered through a loudspeaker. Where it is possible to deliver the sound through earphones, individual ear thresholds can be obtained.

VRA may be used until the child is able to perform pure tone audiometry. It is also sometimes used with pure tone audiometry as the reward, instead of using 'play' techniques.

Cooperative tests (18–30 months)

The age range from eighteen months to two years is a difficult period, where the child is too sophisticated for distraction tests but not ready for pure tone audiometry. The cooperative test makes use of the child's developing understanding of language and is in fact a very simple speech test. It makes use of the child's speech perception in the following way. Children are expected to perform simple instructions, presented at varying known intensities of speech using toys as a stimulus. For example:

- give it to Mummy;
- put it in the box;
- put it on the bed.

It is very important for the tester to establish that all vocabulary used in the test is known to the child. Usually the commands are established at conversational level with additional visual cues available to the child. The tester's voice is then lowered and commands are given out of sight. The quietest response level is measured using a sound level meter.

Performance testing (30 months – 4 years)

In this test the child is conditioned to perform a simple task on hearing the word 'go' (low frequency), and similarly, the stimulus 's' (high frequency). At the command ('go' or 's'), the child must make a response, such as placing a brick in a box or a man in a boat. The child is first taught, or conditioned, to perform this task. Once the child understands the game, the tester moves out of the line of vision and gives the commands. It is important to maintain a constant distance from the child's ear. The voice intensity is measured using a sound level meter. Once a child is conditioned to reliably perform an action in response to a stimulus, it should be possible to undertake pure tone audiometry.

Pure tone audiometry (PTA)

In pure tone audiometry, the test signal is delivered to the outer ear via headphones, which means that each ear can be tested separately. Pure tone audiometry is covered later in this chapter.

Summary of test procedures

The ages given for the various test procedures depend upon the child's stage of development and are therefore approximate:

- 6 months – behavioural observation audiometry;
- 6–18 months – distraction tests;
- 6–36 months – visual response audiometry;

- 18–30 months – cooperative tests;
- 30 months – 4 years – performance tests;
- 4+ years – pure tone audiometry using 'play' techniques;
- 6+ years – pure tone audiometry (conventional).

All these tests require the child being tested to make a response, either an automatic reflex response as in the distraction test or a conditioned response of some type. They also depend upon the tester to make a subjective judgement about that response.

Objective hearing tests

Objective hearing tests are those which do not require the child to make a behavioural response, but merely to cooperate with the test procedures. Responses to the sound stimulus are evoked, monitored and recorded by the equipment used. Responses arise from certain points along the auditory pathway, according to the test. Objective tests in common use include:

- evoked response audiometry;
- otoacoustic emissions;
- tympanometry;
- acoustic (stapedial) reflex testing.

Evoked response audiometry (ERA)

Evoked response audiometry (ERA) involves recording electrical activity evoked by sounds. Responses may be elicited from various places (the ear, the brainstem and the auditory cortex) along the length of the auditory pathway.

Where ERA is used with children, hearing thresholds are most commonly estimated from the brainstem response. The auditory brainstem response (ABR) can be obtained without the need for surgery or anaesthetics. Neural activity, in response to sound signals, is received by electrodes, which are placed on the head. The ABR can be reliably recorded at near threshold levels in the high frequencies, if the child is resting or asleep. However, the results of the test have to be interpreted from the recorded wave-form and information obtained about the hearing loss in the low frequency region is not ideal.

Otoacoustic emissions (OAE) and neo-natal screening

The cochlea creates internal vibrations whenever it processes sound. These internal vibrations are emitted from the ear as very low intensity sounds: otoacoustic emissions. During testing, an acoustic signal is presented to the ear and the following otoacoustic emissions (or 'cochlear echoes') are measured. The presence of an evoked otoacoustic emission indicates normal cochlea and middle ear function.

Otoacoustic emissions are usually evoked using clicks. A probe, or insert earphone, containing a miniature loudspeaker and microphone, is fitted in the ear canal (see Figure 3.2). The miniature loudspeaker delivers a series of clicks to the ear canal, and the miniature microphone picks up the evoked otoacoustic emissions. These are relayed to a computer, which displays the results.

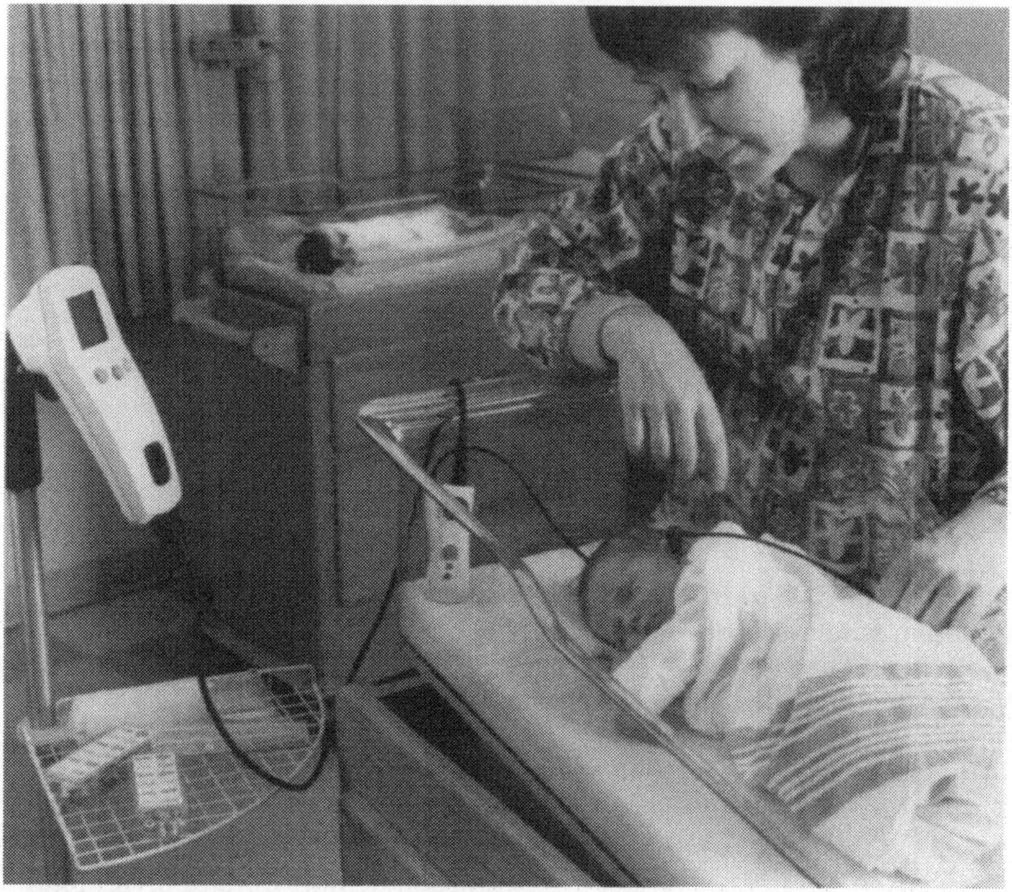

Figure 3.2 Otoacoustic emissions being used to screen the hearing of a new born baby (photograph courtesy of Grason-Stadler Inc)

The presence of emissions usually means normal or near normal hearing around the frequency of the stimulus used to evoke them. Absence of emissions tends to point to possible cochlear damage or middle ear problems but a very small minority of normally hearing people have no recordable emissions.

It is generally accepted that the early detection and management of deafness is important in alleviating delay in the development of communication and related social and emotional development.

Ideally a neonatal screening programme will identify all babies with a significant hearing loss at a very early age and universal screening is the aim. Where universal screening is not possible, babies with an increased risk of hearing loss are usually targeted. These babies are often those in neonatal intensive care units but may also include babies who have a family history of deafness or evidence of congenital syndromes related to deafness.

Clinically evoked otoacoustic emissions are widely used in neonatal screening as the test is non-invasive and takes less than five minutes to perform. Babies who fail to show otoacoustic emissions are followed up with evoked response audiometry.

Tympanometry

A tympanometer is an instrument which provides information on the functioning and status of the middle ear. Tympanometry is an objective test and, as it requires little cooperation, it can be carried out at any age and with any degree of deafness. It allows for the measurement of the elasticity or 'compliance' of the eardrum and the middle ear system.

A low frequency tone is introduced into the ear canal, via an air-tight probe, and at the same time the air pressure in the ear canal is altered. When sound reaches the eardrum, some of it will pass through and some will be reflected. If the middle ear system is stiff, much of the sound will be reflected back from the drum. If the system is elastic, more of the sound will pass through. Thus, changes in the middle ear affect the stiffness, and hence the efficiency, of the system. The ear is most compliant when the air pressure inside middle ear cavity is the same as that in the ear canal. By altering the pressure in the ear canal and studying the proportion of the probe tone that is reflected back, the compliance can be measured. The results are recorded on a tympanogram and show the degree of mobility of the middle ear. Abnormalities in the shape of the tympanogram, together with the pressure recorded, suggest certain middle ear problems, as shown in Figure 3.3. The volume of the ear canal is also noted, as this can show, for example, if the eardrum is perforated.

Acoustic or stapedial reflex testing

Loud sound causes the stapedius muscle in the middle ear to contract and stiffen. This protects the ear by reducing the amount of sound admitted. The acoustic reflex is tested by introducing a sound stimulus, at about 85dB above threshold, to one ear. The muscles in both ears contract and the change can therefore be recorded in either ear. A reflex will not be recorded in an ear that has a significant middle ear problem. Results may also provide information about the hearing loss of the ear

Condition	Pressure	Compliance	Average (cc)	Shape
Normal	Normal	Normal	0.3 – 1.3	
Otosclerosis	Normal	Low	0.1 – 1.01	
Otitis media	Low	Low	0.06 – 0.81	
Discontinuity and scarring	Normal	High (can be normal)	0.76 – 3.66	

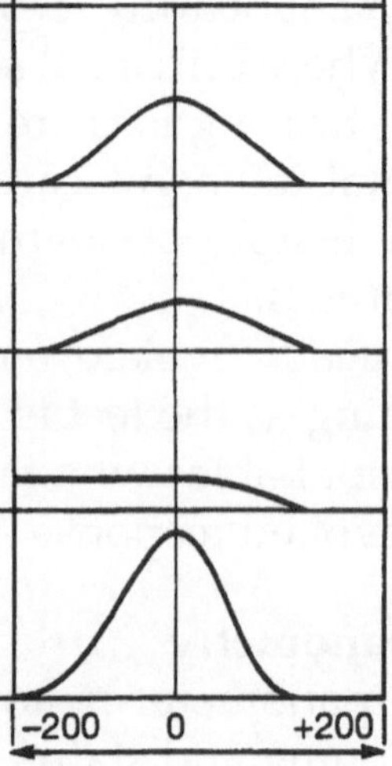

Figure 3.3 Tympanogram results (from Tate 1994, with permission)

receiving the sound stimulus. With a conductive hearing loss, the threshold for the reflex will be raised, for example with a conductive loss of 30dBHL, a reflex would be expected at about 110dBHL. In the case of a sensori-neural hearing loss, the presence of a reflex may indicate an abnormal response to loud sounds (recruitment) which is common with cochlear deafness.

Pure tone audiometry

Pure tone audiometry is the procedure most commonly used for the measurement of degree of deafness. As it normally gives the most detailed and accurate results it should be used as soon as the child can be perform reliably. Young children are taught to perform reliably through conditioning.

Conditioning involves showing the child how they are expected to respond and ensuring the child is responding reliably to a tone they can hear clearly, before commencing the actual test.

Tones of a single frequency (pure tones) are introduced:

- via headphones (air conduction), or
- via a bone vibrator (bone conduction).

Testing by air conduction

The tester selects the frequency and the intensity of the pure tones and presents them through headphones, to each ear in turn, usually in the following order: 1kHz, 2kHz, 4kHz, 8kHz, 500Hz, 250Hz. For young children, with a short attention span, three or four frequencies, often 500Hz, 1kHz and 4kHz, are initially targeted to give an overall picture of hearing levels.

Each tone presentation is brief, about one to three seconds. Tones are presented first at a level that is sufficient for the child to hear clearly. The audiologist uses an agreed method of checking to find the level at which the child can just hear the tone (threshold).

The most common method involves reducing the tone in 10dB steps until the child no longer responds and then raising the level of the tone in 5dB steps until the child responds again. This procedure is often referred to as '10 down and 5 up'. The tone is raised and lowered in this way until the child responds at the same level twice out of a maximum of four times when ascending from the inaudible to the audible. This is then established as the threshold of hearing. The results are plotted on an audiogram (see Chapter 2).

If one ear has a much greater level of hearing loss than the other by air conduction (at least 40dB difference), the sound can cross the head and be heard by the opposite ear. In this case, it is possible that the ear being tested could really be much deafer than it appears to be. Masking must be used if the audiologist wishes to know the true hearing level in the worse ear. This is where a noise is presented to the non-test (better) ear, at required levels to prevent that ear from hearing the test tone. The test tones are presented to the other (worse) ear and the correct thresholds will be obtained.

As an example, if the right ear is dead and the left ear has a hearing loss of 30dB, it could appear that the dead ear is hearing at 70dBHL. When masking noise is introduced to the left ear, it will become apparent that the results are false.

The air conduction part of this test provides an assessment of the degree of deafness but not the nature of the deafness i.e. whether the deafness is sensori-neural or conductive. To establish the nature of the deafness the child is further tested using a bone conduction headband to deliver the sound directly to the inner ear, via the bones of the skull, bypassing the outer and middle ears.

Testing by bone conduction

Testing by bone conduction is carried out in the same way as by air conduction, except that a bone conduction headband is used instead of headphones, with the bone conductor placed on the mastoid bone behind the ear. A smaller range of frequencies (usually 500Hz, 1kHz, 2kHz, 4kHz) is tested, as bone conduction is inaccurate at high and low frequencies.

When testing by bone conduction, the signal travels through the bones of the skull to both ears. Therefore the response to sound will usually be for the better cochlea. Thresholds of hearing gained through bone conduction indicate the level of sensori-neural deafness. The difference between the air conduction result and the bone conduction result is known as the air–bone gap (see Figure 3.4) and this indicates the extent of any conductive hearing loss. If the loss is purely conductive the bone conduction results will be within normal limits.

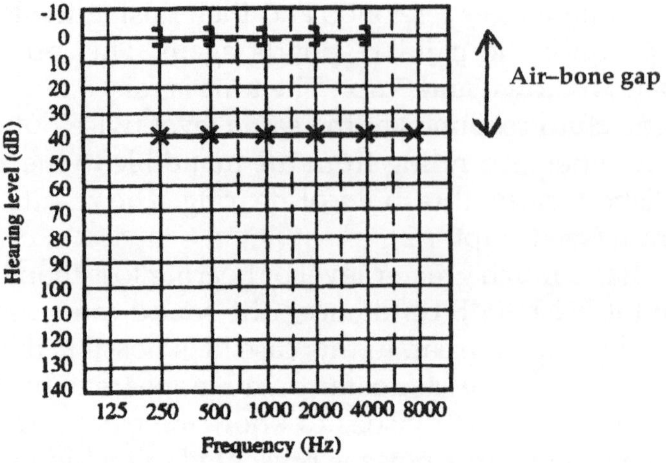

Key: Left
Air conduction, masked if necessary ×
Bone conduction, masked]

Figure 3.4 An audiogram showing an air–bone gap (conductive hearing loss) (diagram courtesy of A&M Hearing Ltd)

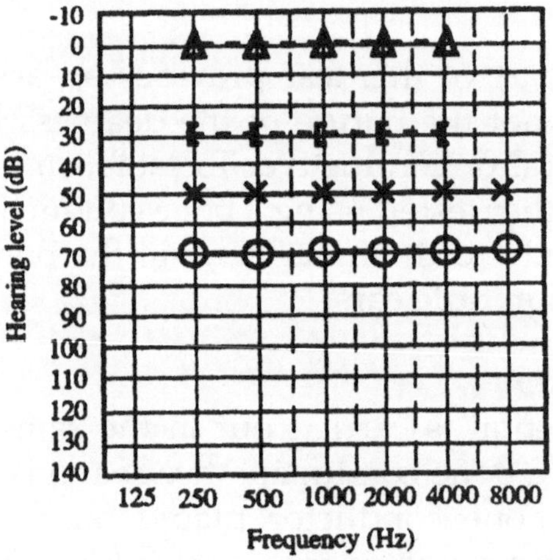

Key:	Right		Left
Air conduction, masked if necessary	○		×
Bone conduction, not masked		△	
Bone conduction, masked	[		]

Figure 3.5 An audiogram showing the appropriate use of symbols (diagram courtesy of A&M Hearing Ltd)

The results by bone conduction are plotted on the same audiogram form (see Figure 3.5) as the air conduction results. The symbol used for bone conduction (not masked) is a triangle, which symbolises that the sound is carried to both ears. Masking must always be used if the audiologist wishes to know the degree of deafness in each ear by bone conduction. The symbol used for masked bone conduction on the audiogram is a square bracket, opening towards the side tested. Each threshold value on the audiogram is joined using a broken line.

Play audiometry

Pure tone audiometry using conventional methods can be applied to adults and older children. 'Play audiometry' is the term used when pure tone testing young children, usually up to the age of about eight years. Conventional methods involve pressing a signal button in response to the test tones. In play audiometry, the child is taught (conditioned) to respond to the test tones by carrying out a specific action, such as putting a ball on a stick or a peg in a board, every time they hear a sound. By treating audiometry as a game, the younger child's concentration is improved and the results obtained are both more reliable and more detailed. Some children as young as two or three can provide reliable and valid thresholds for the experienced audiologist using play techniques.

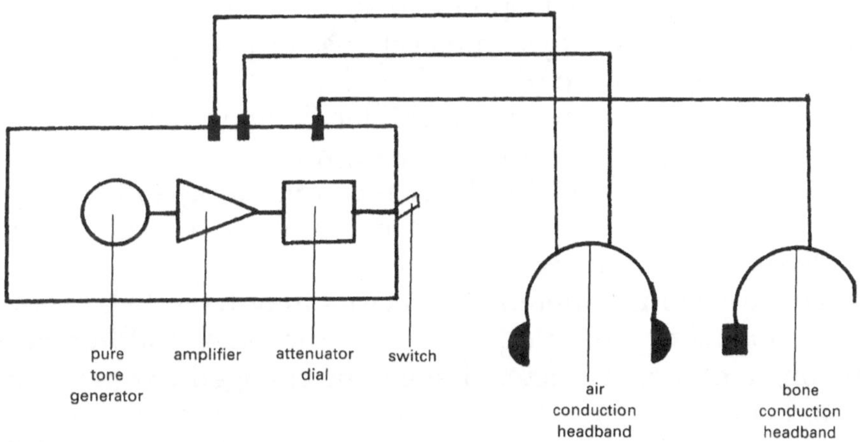

Figure 3.6 The parts of an audiometer (after Tate 1994)

The audiometer

An audiometer (see Figure 3.6), is the technical equipment used to establish the degree of deafness by comparing the individual's hearing levels to average normal hearing levels. It must be highly accurate to be of value and to this end all audiometers have to be calibrated to British Standards when they are new and at least annually thereafter. All audiometers should comply with British Standards (BS5966, 1980).

Assessment of children with complex needs

The National Deaf Children's Society (NDCS 1996) estimate that up to 40 per cent of deaf children will have additional needs, such as visual problems and developmental delay. Children with complex needs are not a homogeneous group; they have atypical or delayed development, which influences the audiologist's ability to use routine tests. Assessment is a challenging and highly specialised area and information from carers takes on heightened importance. Tests used are generally chosen from the battery of tests available, deemed to be most appropriate to the developmental age of the child. Most audiologists see only a very small number of children with complex needs and yet the audiologist has to develop an array of flexible strategies, in order to modify procedures to meet the needs of these children. Examples of such modifications could include:

- Responses to sound may have to be *any* repeatable behaviour that the child makes to sound, for instance kicking, dribbling, pointing, rocking, banging, or even holding breath in.
- 'Eye pointing' (looking towards an object) may be useful with some physically handicapped children as a response, for example in a limited toy test.
- Sounds used to evoke a response may have to be environmental sounds, such as noisy toys, musical instruments, banging doors, television or a cup and spoon.
- Conditioning to sound through visual / tactile re-enforcement, pairing touch or light with presentation of the sound.
- Visual stimuli may be unhelpful when conditioning autistic children and loud noises should be avoided, as these children may be extremely sensitive to sound.
- In distraction testing, different distractors may have to be used, for example bubbles, or a flashing torch. In some cases, children need no distraction, in others distractors have to be changed frequently as the child loses interest.
- Extra response time may be needed, for example dyslexic children often show a long delay between hearing a sound and responding to it.

Objective tests, such as those described earlier in this chapter, may also be appropriate for this group of children, especially where accurate assessment of hearing threshold is not possible. Objective tests do not provide the whole picture and it is important to add behavioural and observational information to those results. Also, in ABR for example, multiply handicapped children often require sedation though they may be less responsive to it. Tympanometry is non-invasive and important in screening for middle ear problems.

Implications for teachers

The diagnosis of deafness does not rely on a single test. With young children it is particularly important that a combination of behavioural and objective tests are carried out. These, together with observational evidence from parents and involved professionals, all contribute to the audiological profile of the individual child.

Newly qualified teachers of the deaf are not expected to be skilled in administering all these tests. Teachers may at some stage and in some areas become involved in testing children at home or in a school or hospital setting.

Teachers need to be aware of all the common testing techniques so that they are able to discuss them, and children's results, with parents and other professionals. It is particularly important that they are able to interpret results of hearing tests and to appreciate the likely implications for language development and learning.

Summary

This chapter has outlined the test procedures commonly used in hospitals and clinics. It has approached them in an approximately developmental order, as it is appropriate to test children's hearing from a developmental rather that a chronological age. It has highlighted the fact that testing has two main aims. Firstly, to screen the population for those children who have a significant hearing loss and, secondly, to diagnose accurately the degree and nature of the loss. Accurate assessment is particularly important for the prescription of amplification systems in order to maximise opportunities for developing speech and language.

Further reading

Coninx, F. and Moore J. (1997) 'The multiply handicapped deaf child', in McCracken, W. and Laiode-Kemp, S. (eds) *Audiology in Education.* London: Whurr Publishers.

McCormick, B. (1993) *Paediatric Audiology. 0-5 years,* 2nd edn. London: Whurr Publishers.

Maltby, M. (2001) Chapter 6, 'The assessment procedure', in *Principles of Hearing Aid Audiology,* 2nd edn. London: Whurr Publishers.

Wiley, T. L. and Fowler, C. G. (1997) *Acoustic Immittance Measures.* San Diego: Singular Publishing Group.

Chapter 4

Amplification Systems

Hearing aids

Amplification systems (hearing aids) are designed to enhance the auditory experience of hearing impaired people. For children, the quality of this experience is important as without effective exposure to the sounds of the environment and particularly of speech the opportunity to develop spoken language will be diminished.

Hearing aids cannot restore normal hearing. The problems here are:

- The hearing aid provides only a limited frequency range and there is inevitably some distortion of the sound.
- Sensori-neural hearing loss creates reduced discrimination and difficulty in separating speech from noise, in addition to reducing hearing.

Hearing aids attempt to redress the problems with differing (limited) degrees of success. Separation of speech from background noise remains the greatest challenge to hearing aid manufacturers.

Although hearing aids will not restore a child's hearing to normal, they can provide experience of sound that would otherwise remain unheard. All deaf children should be encouraged to wear their hearing aids. This is to ensure that they are given the maximum opportunity to fully utilise their residual hearing. In the early days it will require a great deal of support, encouragement and management from parents and teachers to develop the skills of listening. Given support and encouragement from the beginning, most deaf children and adults wear their hearing aids happily and gain benefit from them. The degree of benefit will depend upon the hearing aid, its fitting and the hearing loss itself.

How the hearing aid works

It is important to have a basic understanding of how a hearing aid works, in order to:

- ensure that hearing aids are working at maximum efficiency;
- support the establishment and management of hearing aid wearing in young deaf children.

Although technology changes very quickly, in general, all hearing aids consist of the same basic components (see Figure 4.1). These are:

- a microphone which picks up sound from the environment and transduces (changes) it into an electrical signal;
- an amplifier which increases the electrical signal;
- the power supply which comes from the battery, provides the energy for the increase in sound output;
- the volume control which adjusts the level of amplification;
- a receiver or 'loudspeaker' of the hearing aid;
- an earmould which connects the receiver to the wearer's ear.

The microphone

The microphone may be omnidirectional or directional. Omnidirectional microphones are the commonly used microphones. They have one entrance (known as a port) for sound waves. This usually faces forward to receive sound mainly from the front.

Directional microphones usually have two entrances, or ports, for sound. One of these faces forward, whilst the other faces to the rear. It is usually the case that the listener wishes to hear sound from in front. Sound from behind tends to be unwanted noise. In order to give prominence to sound from the front, sound entering the rear port is delayed very slightly.

The reason for this delay is as follows:

- Since sound waves radiate in all directions, sounds from the rear will enter by both the rear and the forward facing ports.
- If the delay built in is such that these sound waves arrive at opposite sides of the diaphragm at the same time, they will cancel each other out (as with phase cancellation, see Chapter 2).
- Sound from the front will be heard more clearly than from the back.

Directional microphones offer a small degree of extra benefit over omnidirectional microphones, although not in all situations, e.g. not if listening to music.

Probably the most important time for a directional microphone to be fitted is if it is only possible for a child to use one hearing aid despite deafness in both ears (bilateral hearing loss).

The amplifier

The amplifier (see Figure 4.1) can be considered a control device. The amplifier will be selected by the manufacturer to amplify over a certain frequency range and to provide a certain power output. All hearing aids have some element of signal processing and attempt to 'shape' the sound output. This is reflected in the frequency response of the hearing aid.

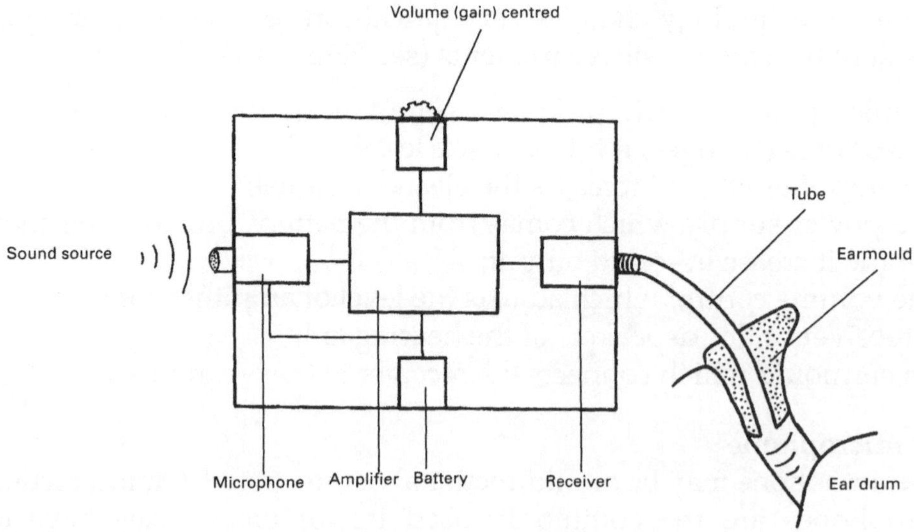

Figure 4.1 The basic components of a hearing aid system (after Tate 1994)

Modifications can be made by the audiologist to reduce the output of the aid (to avoid sounds being too loud) and to further shape the frequency response according to the hearing loss. The output of the aid can be reduced by output limiting, which simply cuts off the output at a particular point, or compression, which compresses the whole signal (see Figure 4.2). The aim of shaping the frequency response is generally to 'mirror' the audiogram, and thus to provide appropriate amplification, e.g. the greatest amplification where the loss is greatest.

This further shaping of the sound signal is achieved by:

- trimmer controls on the hearing aid which are adjusted with a screwdriver, or
- a computer programming link to the hearing aid.

Power supply

The power supply for almost all hearing aids is a battery. The only exceptions are speech training units and group hearing aids (see Chapter 5) which may be mains powered.

The battery current requirements of different hearing aids vary widely and therefore the battery life can vary widely from one aid to another. An estimate of battery life should be provided when a hearing aid is fitted.

Batteries are of different types and available in many sizes. However, most hearing aids use a battery 'pill'; the smaller the hearing aid, the smaller the 'pill'. These days most battery 'pills' are of the zinc-air type. These have a number of air holes on the top side, which are covered until

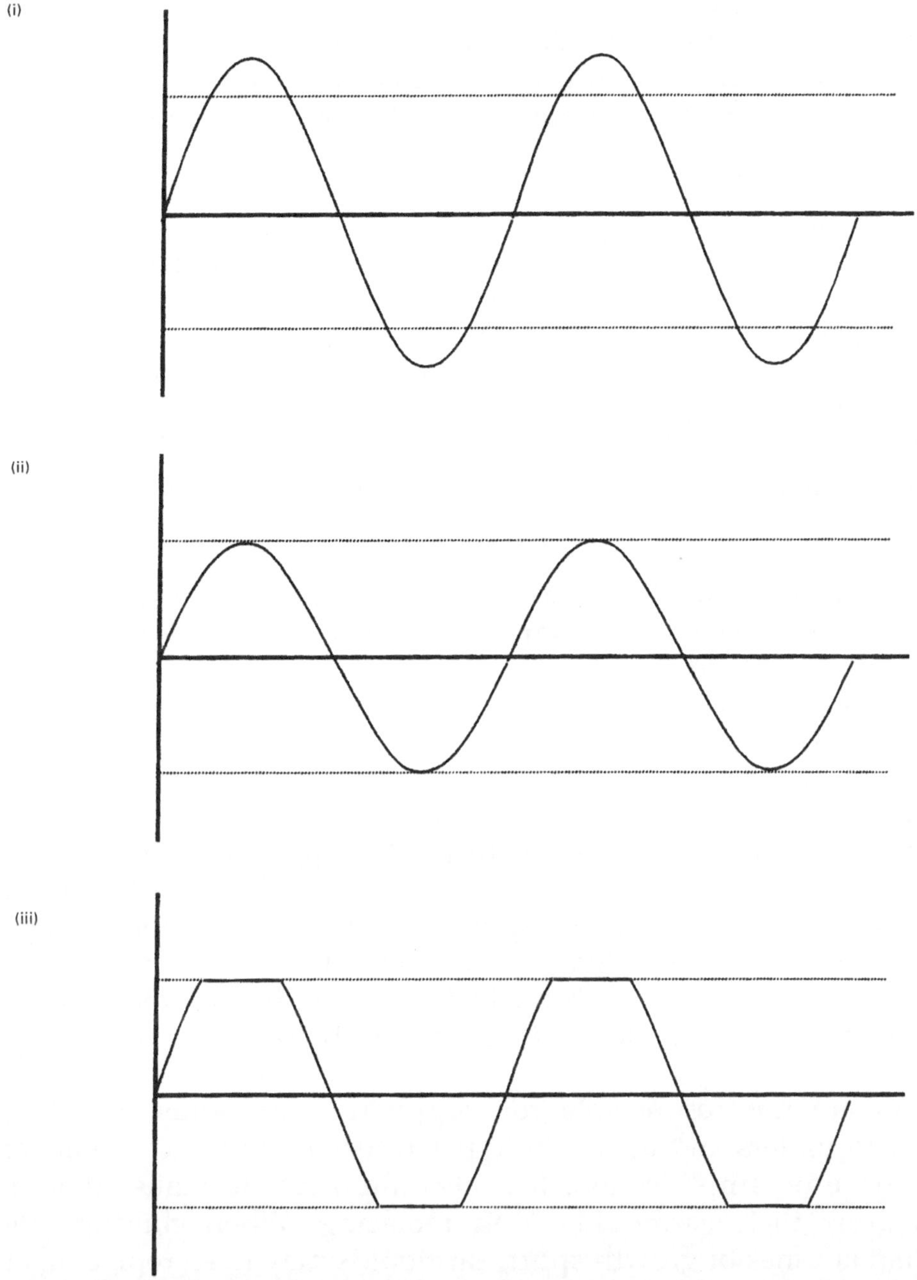

Figure 4.2 Compression and output limiting: (i) the full signal; (ii) the signal with compression; (iii) the signal with output limiting

the battery is required. When the cover (a small adhesive tab) is removed, the battery starts to draw oxygen from the air and its chemical process begins. Once the tab has been removed, replacing the tab cannot stop the chemical process.

These batteries tend to run out with very little warning. It is therefore important to know how long the battery will last in the particular hearing aid and to change it before it runs out. Small children often cannot tell the teacher that their aid is not working and may go for a full day with a dead battery, if routine changing is not carried out.

Rechargeable batteries are commonly used for radio hearing aids (see Chapter 5).

The volume control

The volume control (or gain control) is usually a serrated dial or wheel, which adjusts the level of amplification.

The amount of increase is not steady (linear) over the full turn of the dial. It tends to be the case that most of the gain, about 70 per cent, is delivered turning the volume control only halfway on. Turning the volume control 'full on' provides only a limited amount of extra gain and is likely to distort the sound. Some hearing aids control the volume automatically.

The receiver

A receiver (see Figure 4.1) is a loudspeaker or a microphone in reverse. It converts the amplified electrical signal back to sound which is relayed to the ear via the earmould.

The frequency response of the hearing aid is further shaped by the receiver and by the earmould.

The earmould

An earmould connects the receiver to the hearing aid wearer and is manufactured to fit the individual ear. The earmould is a weak link in the hearing aid system, however appropriate the amplification. If the earmould is not effectively fitted in the ear, acoustic feedback will occur.

Acoustic feedback is the high pitched whistling heard when sound leaks from the earmould and is picked up by the microphone and re-amplified.

Teachers are not responsible for supplying earmoulds but it is important to understand about the types of ear mould and the effect they can have on amplification. It is also important to realise that as children grow their earmoulds need replacing. When children are young, and at times of growth spurt, earmoulds may need replacing at very frequent intervals. An earmould which is too small, or which is not a good fit, will inevitably feedback, introducing distortion and also discomfort for the wearer and others to whom the whistling is audible.

Earmoulds need to provide a good seal in the ear to prevent feedback. An earmould will only be as good as the ear impression from which it is made. The audiologist should make impressions using a silicone-based material and following an approved technique (BSA 1986). Basically, a foam or cotton wool block or 'tamp' is inserted well down the ear canal, just past the second bend. Postaural aids, if these are to be used, should then be placed over the ears. These aids will alter the ear shape and this must be reflected in the shape of the impression. The impression material is syringed into the ear and left to set, without being pressed flat, which would distort the impression.

The type of finished earmould will be chosen according to the type of hearing aid. For a body-worn aid, the earmould has to be solid and fitted with a ring and clip, which will attach it to the receiver of the body-worn aid.

An earmould for a post-aural, or behind-the-ear, hearing aid will be fitted with a tube to attach it to the tone hook or 'elbow' of the aid. Earmoulds for this kind of hearing aid can be obtained in a wide variety of styles (see Figure 4.3) and materials, although the choice is to some extent restricted by the degree of the hearing loss and by the size of the ear. Soft materials tend to be used for young children and those who are severely or profoundly deaf, because they are less likely to cause damage to the ear in the course of rough play. Also, they tend to seal more tightly in the ear. However soft materials are best used in 'shell' (solid) moulds and acrylic material may be preferred by older children as it is available in more cosmetically acceptable shapes. Acrylics may be hard or 'soft' (this is quite hard but softens somewhat as it warms in the ear). Soft acrylic is generally preferable to hard acrylic for children.

Types of hearing aid

Hearing aids come in a variety of shapes and sizes. Most commonly they are worn in or behind the ear. Types of hearing aids include:

- post-aural or behind the ear (BTE);
- spectacle;
- in the ear (ITE);
- body worn (BW);
- transposition;
- bone conduction;
- bone anchored;
- vibro-tactile;
- cochlear implants (see Chapter 7).

Most hearing aids use air conduction; that is, the sound passes directly from the hearing aid through the air into the ear canal. Other methods of conduction are used in bone conduction hearing aids, cochlear implants and vibro-tactile aids.

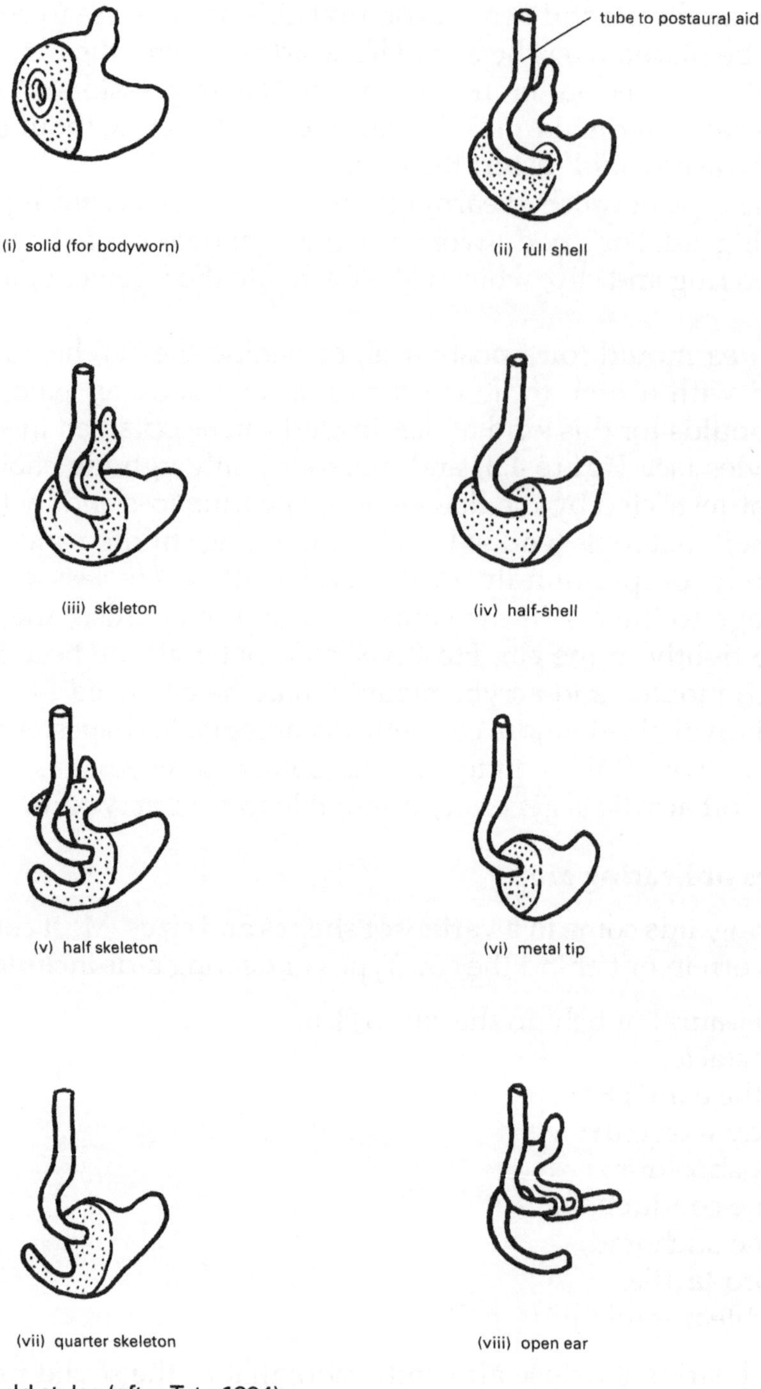

Figure 4.3 Earmould styles (after Tate 1994)

Post-aural hearing aids

Post-aural aids are the most commonly prescribed aids for deaf children. They are available in a wide variety of sizes and colours (see Figure 4.4) and can be fitted successfully to almost every hearing loss. Post-aural hearing aids are also known as behind-the-ear (BTE) hearing aids.

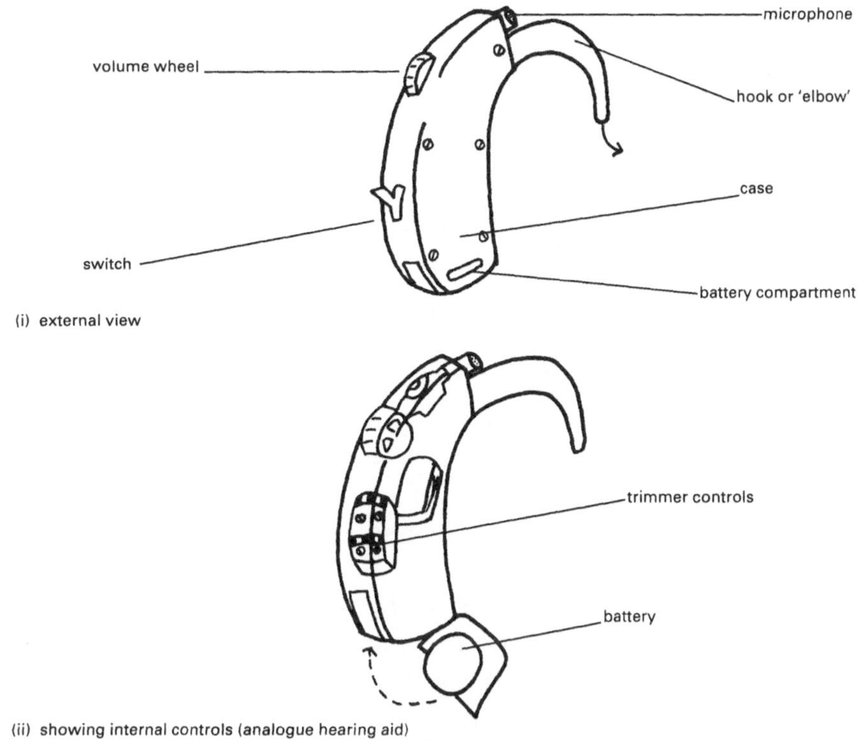

Figure 4.4 A post-aural or behind-the-ear (BTE) hearing aid

Post-aural aids have all the components housed in a case, which is worn behind the ear. The aid is linked to an earmould by a tube. Most post-aural aids have a forward-facing microphone as most of the desired sound comes from the front. Children should wear two hearing aids whenever possible and appropriate. Two hearing aids have the advantage of reproducing the auditory input binaurally. Binaural advantages include:

- ability to hear from both sides
- ability to localise sound
- enhanced ability to discriminate speech in noise
- less distortion
- improved sound quality
- increased loudness without increased amplification.

Air conduction spectacle aids

Spectacle aids (Figure 4.5) are basically post-aural aids attached to, or built within, the arm of the spectacle. The aid is linked to the ear canal by a tube and earmould. These aids are designed to overcome the problem of space and comfort when wearing both spectacles and hearing aids at the same time.

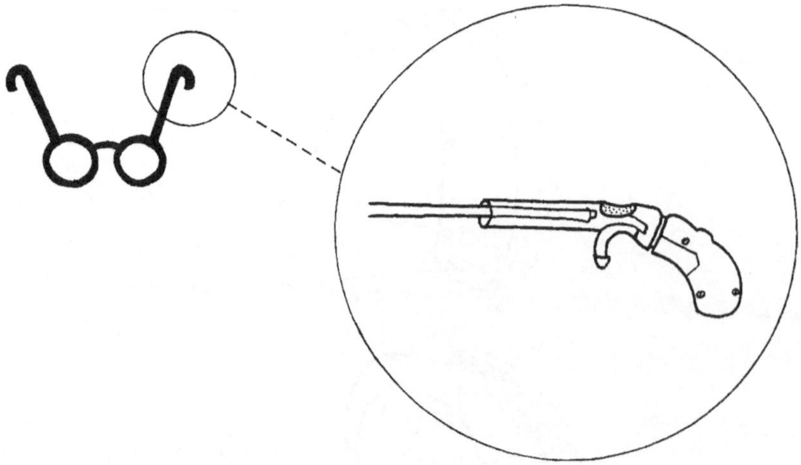

Figure 4.5 An air conduction spectacle hearing aid

In-the-ear hearing aids

These are aids where all the components of the hearing aid are fitted in the earmould itself. In theory, in-the-ear hearing aids can provide amplification for all losses apart from the most severe and profound. However, the size of children's ears restricts the size of the aid and so the amount of gain and output possible. There is also an increased likelihood of acoustic feedback as the microphone and receiver are in very close proximity. The major disadvantage of in-the-ear aids for children is that the 'shell' or casing has to be replaced as the child grows.

In-the-ear (ITE) hearing aids (see Figure 4.6) for children will tend to be full shell, but with larger ears, it is possible to have smaller ITEs, that are placed mainly or completely in the ear canal. These are known as canal aids. There are also very tiny hearing aids which are hidden completely in the canal (CIC hearing aids), these are very unlikely to be used by children.

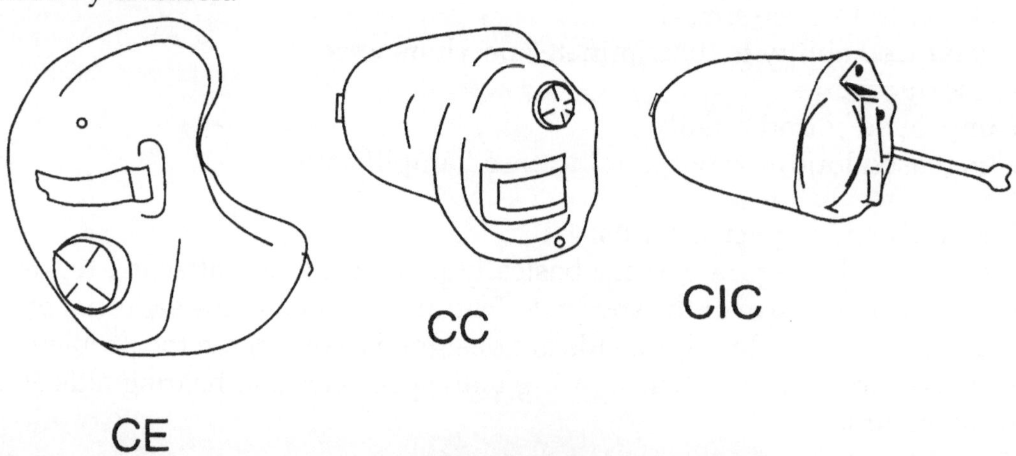

Figure 4.6 Styles of in-the-ear (ITE) hearing aids (diagram courtesty of Starkey Laboratories Ltd)

Body worn aids

In a body worn hearing aid (see Figure 4.7) the microphone, amplifier and batteries are contained in a hearing aid case, which is linked by a cord or 'lead' to an external receiver and earmould. Body worn aids are relatively bulky. Body-worn aids are not widely used for children, except for those with special needs for whom the larger sized controls may be easier to handle. The hearing aid case needs to be positioned high up on the chest and is often worn in a harness. The cord linking the aid to the receiver in the ear may be single or a Y-cord. The Y-cord allows for input into both ears but does not reflect true binaural hearing because there is only one sound input. Two body-worn aids are therefore the preferred choice where body worn aids are prescribed for a deaf child.

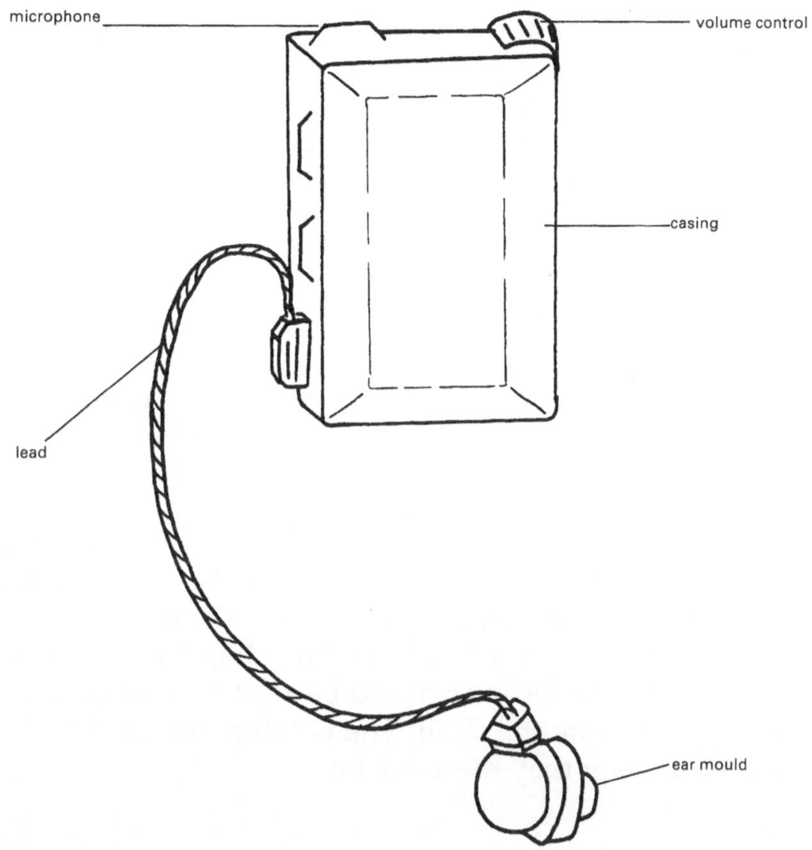

Figure 4.7 A body-worn hearing aid

The larger size of body-worn aids allows for increased gain and output and a good low frequency response. The separation of microphone and receiver means there is less likelihood of acoustic feedback. The position of the microphone high up on the chest provides good reproduction of the child's own voice but does not allow much separation of the hearing aids, therefore limiting the degree of binaural advantage possible.

The leads and the microphone are vulnerable components. The microphone must not be covered by clothes as these will rub against it making a noise which will interfere with hearing other sounds. The position of the microphones is such that they may easily become blocked by dropped food. A special 'baby cover', obtainable from the hearing aid manufacturer, will solve this problem. The leads from body-worn hearing aids are also particularly vulnerable, not least because children tend to chew or play with them.

Transposition aids

Transposition aids are air conduction hearing aids, either post-aural or body-worn, which aim to address the problem of amplification for hearing losses where there is little or no response to high frequency sounds. High frequency sounds are 'transposed' or shifted into a lower frequency band, which is within the hearing range of the particular person. The frequency band is compressed to maintain the natural structure of the speech signal as far as possible. Intensive auditory training is required to recognise the new transposed signal and to obtain maximum benefit from it.

Bone conduction aids

Bone conduction aids (see Figure 4.8) transmit the amplified sound signal to the cochlea, by mechanically vibrating the bones of the skull. Bone conduction serves to bypass the outer and middle ears. Bone conduction aids have a poor high frequency response. They are used for those conductive hearing problems where the ear cannot be blocked by an earmould, for example, where the ear discharges, or where the child has been born with a malformed or absent external ear.

The bone conduction receiver is attached to a headband and is placed on the mastoid bone. The receiver has to be relatively large to produce sufficient energy to vibrate the skull. The hearing aid used to drive the bone conduction receiver may therefore be:

- body-worn,
- a powerful post-aural or
- a bone conduction spectacle aid.

Bone anchored hearing aids (BAHA)

The BAHA, is a bone conduction hearing aid which is attached to the bone by means of an implanted titanium screw. The aid consists of:

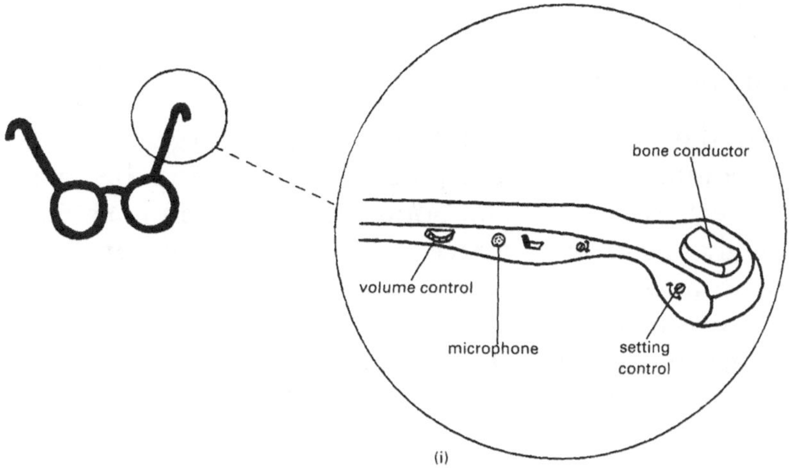

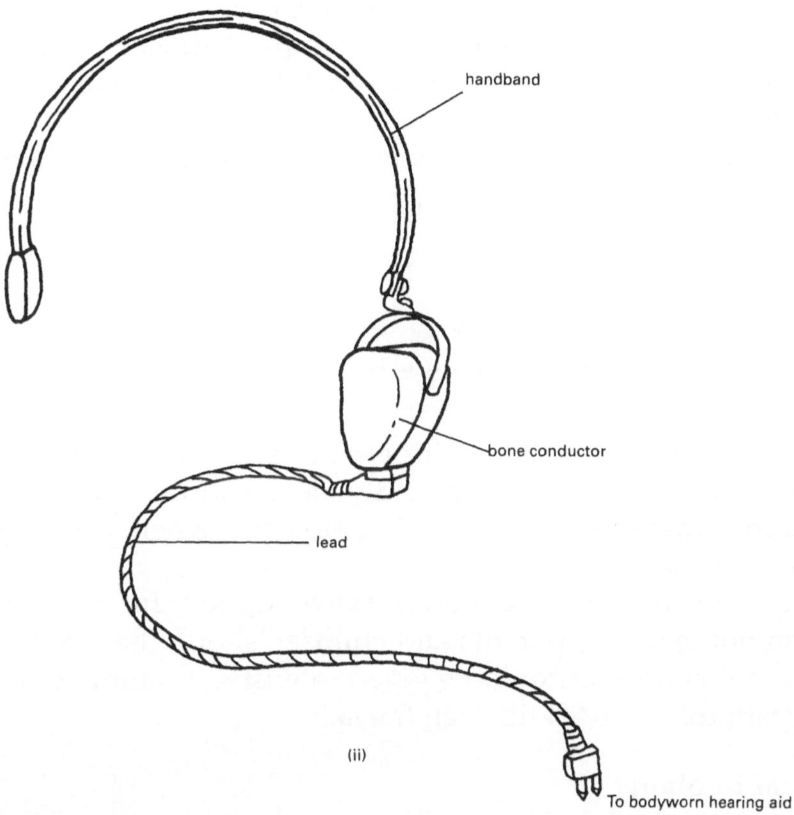

Figure 4.8 Bone conduction hearing aids
(i) Bone conduction spectacles
(ii) Bone conduction headband to be attached to a body worn hearing aid. A similar headband can be driven by a powerful post-aural hearing aid.

- a titanium screw;
- an abutment;
- a hearing aid and insert.

The screw and the abutment are fitted during surgery and time is allowed for osseointegration to take place. The insert and the hearing aid are removable parts of the system. Sound transmission is better with a BAHA because there is direct contact with the bone. Bone anchored aids tend to be more comfortable than conventional bone conduction aids and are certainly more cosmetic, since no headband is required. The main disadvantages are the need for operations and the care and maintenance required. Daily cleaning around the abutment is necessary to prevent infection.

Vibro-tactile aids

These aids transmit information about acoustic signals to the skin. They are usually worn on the wrist. The simplest devices provide limited information through a single channel while more sophisticated devices use multiple channels.

The limited information available through tactile aids includes:

- presence and absence of sound;
- duration of sounds;
- intensity and rhythm;
- length and speed of delivery;
- presence or absence of voicing and
- some pitch information.

These aids may be used on their own or as an addition to hearing aids. They may be useful for profoundly deaf children who receive very limited information through hearing aids and where cochlear implants are not appropriate.

A vibro-tactile aid is a non-invasive option for profoundly deaf children but teachers, parents and children should have realistic expectations, and children should be given intensive training to interpret the tactile patterns received through the skin.

Cochlear implants

Cochlear implants (see Chapter 7) are a type of hearing aid that includes internal and external components. The internal part of the system is implanted in the skull. The external part includes a sound processor.

Analogue versus digital hearing aids

Traditional hearing aids use analogue signal processing. Digital hearing aids are a development of the 1990s and are becoming increasingly important. Teachers are likely to be working with both analogue and digital hearing aids for the foreseeable future but further developments will concentrate on digital signal processing.

Analogue signals use physical variables, such as voltage, to represent the signal. Sound is difficult to amplify and process directly. It is therefore converted to an analogue electrical signal (that is an electrical signal with the same wave form as the original sound) before it is processed. The electrical signal is amplified, the frequency response is adjusted and there may be other processing, for example noise reduction. After the signal has been processed, it is converted back to sound.

Digital signals allow mathematical techniques to be used in processing the signal. Digital means numerical. The incoming sound is converted into an encoded series of numbers, which represent the sound wave. Amplification and filtering are then carried out by digital calculations. In effect, the digital hearing aid is using a computer to process the signal. Signal processing can be carried out by analogue or digital means but digital signal processing (DSP) provides far greater flexibility. Complex processing means that the digital hearing aid can, for example:

- facilitate accurate programming while the aid is being worn;
- adapt continuously to differing situations;
- amplify selectively in different frequency bands;
- reduce the impact of background noise;
- automatically suppress feedback;
- use a fully automatic volume control (with no volume wheel);
- use advanced 'compression' to reduce over-loud signals while increasing very quiet signals.

Figure 4.9 (a) shows sampling points; (b) shows how the waveform appears smoother as more sampling points are taken. In reality, a great number of sampling points are used to create a smooth waveform.

A digital hearing aid is programmed via a personal computer or a dedicated programming unit. A personal computer can be used to programme many different types of digital hearing aids using software known as 'NOAH' and a 'HI-PRO' interface which connects the hearing aid to the computer.

All digital hearing aids are programmable. This simply means that digital programming is used to adjust the hearing aid's parameters. Early programmable hearing aids were not fully digital but were analogue hearing aids, which were programmed digitally.

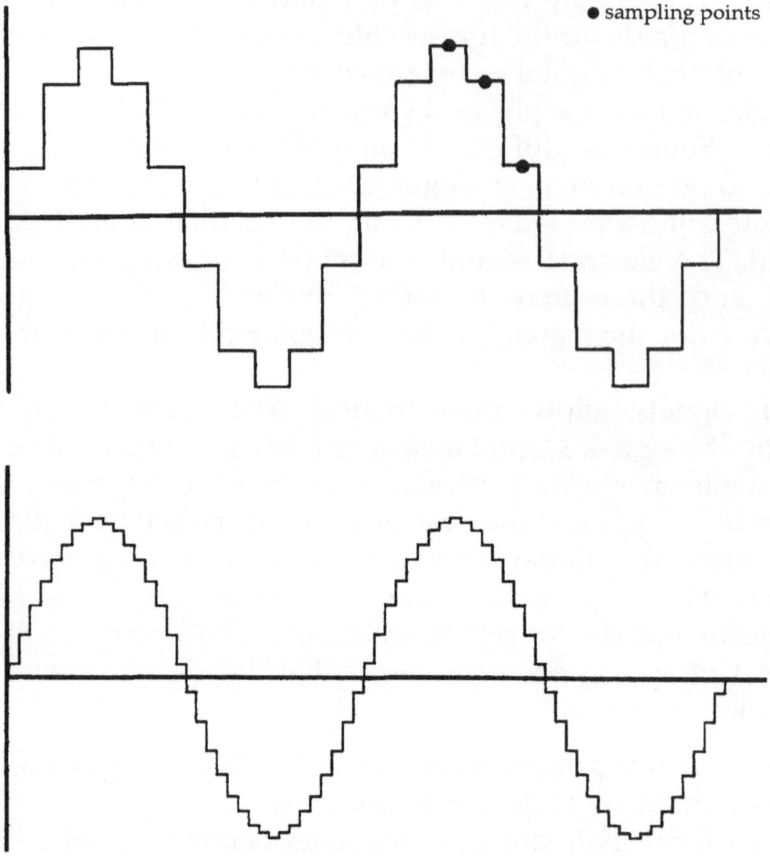

(a)

(b)

Figure 4.9 Digital wave forms
(a) sampling points
(b) the waveform appears smoother as more sampling points are taken. In reality, a great number of sampling points is used to create a smooth waveform

Summary

All teachers of the deaf and those who work with deaf children need to be familiar with types of hearing aids and how they work. This chapter describes:

- how a hearing aid works;
- the different types of hearing aids.

Further reading

Bess, F. H. *et al.* (eds) (1996) *Amplification for Children with Auditory Deficits.* Nashville, Tennessee: Bill Wilkerson Center Press.

DeConde Johnson, C. *et al.* (1997). Chapter 6, 'Amplification and classroom hearing technology', in *Educational Audiology Handbook.* San Diego: Singular Publishing Group.

McCracken, W. (1997) 'Tactile aids', in McCracken W. and Laoide-Kemp S. (eds.) *Audiology in Education.* London: Whurr Publishers.

Plant, G. and Spens, K. E. (1995) Part 1: 'Tactile aids', in *Profound Deafness and Speech Communication.* London: Whurr Publishers.

Maltby, M. (2001). Chapter 5, 'The Hearing Aid System', Chapter 7, 'Hearing Aids and their Performance', Chapter 8, 'Selection and Fitting' and Chapter 9, 'Earmoulds', in *Principles of Hearing Aid Audiology,* 2nd edn. London: Whurr Publishers.

Tate, M. (ed.) (1994) *The Earmould, Current Practice and Technology,* 2nd edn. Hearing Aid Audiology Group, British Society of Audiology, Reading.

Chapter 5

The Acoustic Environment

An acoustically good environment is crucial for effective classroom listening. An acoustically good environment can be defined as one that provides conditions in which useful sounds can be clearly distinguished, and in which noise is suppressed. It is important to understand the conditions under which children are working during the school day, as speech intelligibility is greatly affected by noise and reverberation. Most schools provide an acoustically hostile environment that particularly disadvantages hearing aid wearers.

Factors within the acoustic environment affecting speech intelligibility

Noise

School classrooms tend to be noisy places. Background noise is present even when a classroom is unoccupied. Background noise comes not only from children and adults, both inside and outside the classroom, but also from other sources such as central heating, toilets, traffic, lawn mowers and so on.

When a room is occupied, the background noise level increases. A low 'occupied noise level' is desirable, ideally not more than 45 dBA for classes in which deaf children are to be taught. In practice, this is rarely achieved in classrooms. In mainstream schools, levels of 60 dBA and above are much more common. Noise levels can be much higher in some areas outside the classroom, such as the dining room, and also in classes where classroom control is poor. Background noise can prevent the child from hearing the teacher's voice clearly.

Signal-to-noise ratio

The teacher's voice is usually the signal we wish the child to hear and as such it is not considered as part of the background noise. It is very important that the child can hear the teacher's voice (the signal) above the background noise. The difference between the signal and the background noise is known as the signal-to-noise (S/N) ratio. Signal–to-noise ratios are recorded in dB. (No suffix is used).

For example:

- If the occupied noise level in the classroom is 60dBA and the speech signal is 70dBA, the signal-to-noise ratio is +10dB.
- If the occupied noise level in the classroom is 60dBA and the speech signal is also 60dBA, the signal-to-noise ratio is 0dB.
- If the speech signal remains at 60dBA and the noise level increases to 70dBA then the signal to noise ratio is –10dB.

It is generally accepted by audiologists (Berg 1993, Carr 1997, Flexer 1999) that signal-to-noise ratio is a crucial factor in the deaf child's development of spoken language. Deaf children need a higher signal-to-noise ratio than normally hearing children. They need a signal-to-noise ratio of at least +20dB but this is rarely achieved in the classroom. It is more common to find a ratio of around +5dB.

Wearing a hearing aid tends not to improve the signal-to-noise ratio because hearing aids amplify background noise as well as the signal, although digital hearing aids are able to 'recognise' and reduce some types of background noise.

Speech energy loss

Sound energy decreases as the distance from the source increases. The greater the distance between the source and the listener, the weaker the sound signal and therefore the quieter the sound. Children who are seated close to the teacher can be expected to receive about 80 per cent of the speech signal, while those at the back of the class are likely to receive only about 60 per cent. The point at which the energy level of the speech signal becomes the same as the energy level of the background noise (that is when the signal-to-noise ratio is 0dB) is said to be at the 'critical distance'. Children who have normal hearing and no other learning disadvantage may have sufficient linguistic ability to understand the speech message at a greater distance from the teacher. However, a child with hearing problems will need to hear at a very close distance from the teacher to minimise difficulty with speech recognition.

Direct and reflected sound

Direct sound is that which travels directly from the source to the listener without being reflected off any surfaces. In an open environment, sound will only pass directly to the listener, becoming weaker the further it travels. As shown in Figure 5.1, direct sound intensity decreases 6dB every time the distance from the speaker is doubled. This is known as the inverse square law. For example, if the teacher's voice level at 1 metre away is 60dBA, at 2 metres the sound level will be 54dBA and at 4 metres it will be 48dBA.

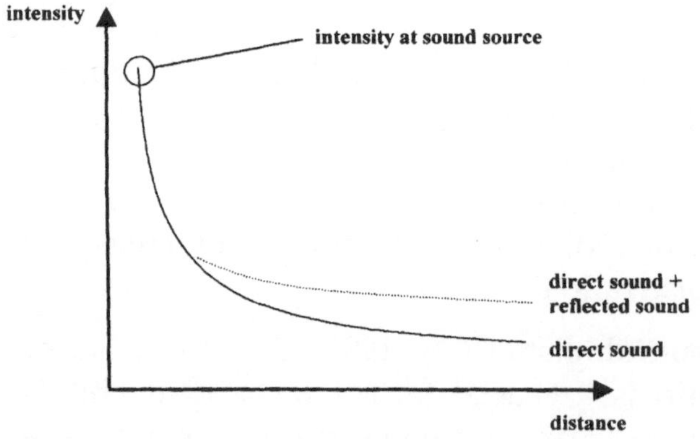

Figure 5.1 Reflections of the direct sound add to the overall level of the sound signal

In an enclosed space however, such as a classroom, the direct sound of the teacher's voice is reflected back from hard objects and surfaces in the room, and absorbed by soft surfaces. The degree to which sound is reflected and absorbed depends on the acoustic characteristics of the environment. The direct sound can be enhanced by reflected sound if it reaches the listener close to the original signal. Reflected sound with a longer delay will smear the direct signal and negatively affect speech intelligibility. Reflected sound with a very long delay can be heard as an echo.

Reverberation

Reverberation is caused by repeated and extended reflection of sounds and has the effect of sound persisting in a room. High frequency sounds tend to be absorbed quickly, while low frequency sounds continue to be reflected.

The time taken for reflected sound to fall by 60 dB (for example to fall from 95dBA to 35dBA) is called the 'reverberation time'. The recommended reverberation time for classrooms in which deaf children are taught is no greater than 0.4 seconds. Many classrooms are much more reverberant than this. The greatest effect of increased reverberation is that the vowel sounds will drown out or 'mask' the consonant sounds, thus reducing speech intelligibility. Reverberation times should ideally be uniform for all speech sounds, not, for example low for vowel sounds (low frequencies) but high for consonant sounds (high frequencies).

In speech, consonant sounds are the weaker higher frequency sounds and vowels are stronger lower frequency sounds. In adverse acoustic conditions, vowels are heard much more readily than consonants. This is particularly unfortunate because consonants only contribute about 10% to the energy of the speech signal but 90% to intelligibility, whilst, on the other hand, vowels contribute about 90% to energy but only 10% to intelligibility (see Figure 5.2).

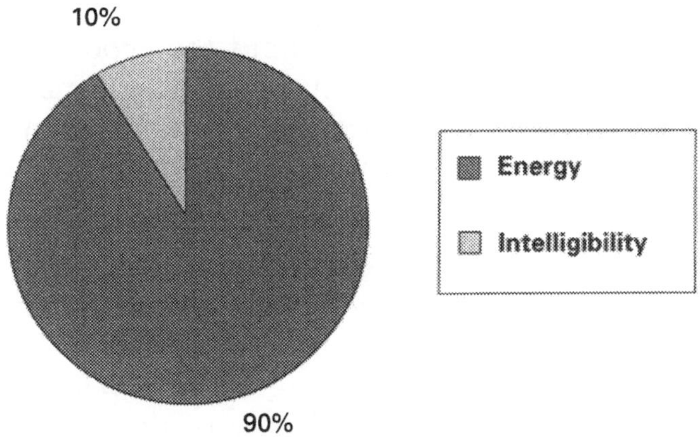

Figure 5.2 The contribution of vowels to the speech signal

Controlling the acoustic environment

Sound treatment in classrooms

There are two major types of noise in the classroom:

- external noise (e.g. from traffic, central heating systems, etc.);
- internal noise (e.g. from children talking, scraping chairs, banging and shuffling, etc.).

External noise is best dealt with at the planning stage. Careful planning of the school building away from external noise sources, such as traffic, can reduce excessive noise. If left to a later stage, it is difficult to reduce external noise significantly and any alterations, such as double-glazing (with a wide gap between the glass panes to insulate against noise), tend to be expensive.

Internal noise is, to a great extent, caused by the pupils. Some measures to reduce internal noise are planning issues, for example, internal noise tends to be greater in open plan classrooms than traditional classrooms.

The adverse effects of reverberation are often improved by installing acoustic (sound absorbent) materials in the classroom. However, absorbent materials tend to absorb high frequency sounds to a much greater extent than low frequencies. Carpets and ceiling tiles, for example, are about five times more absorbent of high frequency sounds than of low frequency sounds. Often these are the only acoustic materials in the classroom. Carpets are useful for suppressing noise from feet, chairs etc. but to be most effective, acoustic treatment should use different absorbent materials to balance absorption across the important speech frequencies. The floor and back wall of the classroom should ideally be sound treated. However, in general, reflected sound from the ceiling and side walls tends to have a positive rather than a negative effect.

The teacher's role

Teachers of the deaf need to be clear about the acoustic, physical and social management of any classrooms in which deaf pupils are educated. It is also part of their role to ensure that all mainstream teachers are familiar with basic strategies for management of the acoustic environment.

- *Noise control:* Noise must be controlled so that it does not interfere with listening. Noise from outside will be transmitted through walls, windows and doors. Noise from outside and inside will interfere with the speech signal. Noise masks the signal, reverberation smears the signal and distance reduces the intensity of the signal. The teacher needs to be aware of acoustical problems in order to facilitate classroom listening.
- *Classroom control:* Internally generated noise is highest when classroom control is poor. If all the pupils are talking and making general noise, the noise level may be as high as 90dBA. Large classes tend to be noisier than small classes but it is the teacher's responsibility to maintain discipline and cooperation and thus reduce noise levels. Ensuring only one person talks at a time, for example, will reduce noise and make it easier for the deaf child to follow. The teacher also needs to make sure that lessons are structured and that visual cues are provided (see Chapter 11).
- *Pupil seating:* The deaf child's seating position in the classroom is important (see Figure 5.3). The child should be comfortably near to the teacher, away from obvious noise sources (such as the door or window), and with an unobstructed view to facilitate lip-reading.
- *Hearing aid management:* Alternative approaches to improve the listening situation rely upon hearing aid technology, for example sound field systems. The signal-to-noise ratio is greatly improved where the teacher speaks closely into a microphone, as the short microphone distance minimises the effects of both noise and reverberation. A constant level of sound can be delivered to the whole class via a sound field system or to the individual deaf child through a radio hearing aid or other amplification system (see Chapter 6).
- *Teaching style:* Teachers need to ensure that their lessons are clearly structured and that the topic or subject is introduced immediately. It helps if the topic and progression through the lesson are reinforced by the written form. Teachers should remain facing the class as much as possible and should speak clearly but at a normal volume and a natural pace. Deaf pupils gain a lot of information from the rhythm and intonation of running speech. Teachers should avoid long periods of unsupported listening time and information should be supported by

visual materials such as diagrams, concept maps and key words. Teachers should avoid using whole-class sessions to correct speech, to encourage repetition or to improve the spoken input from deaf children.

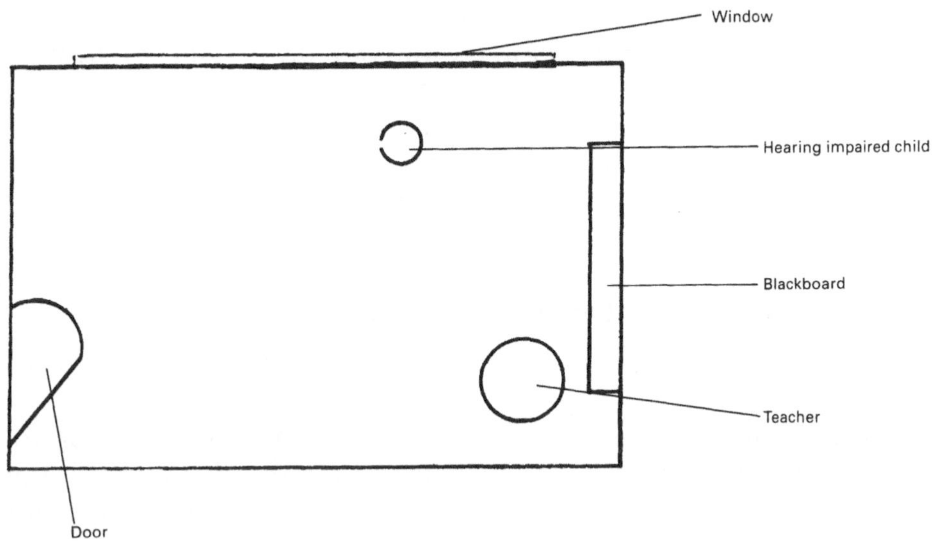

(a)

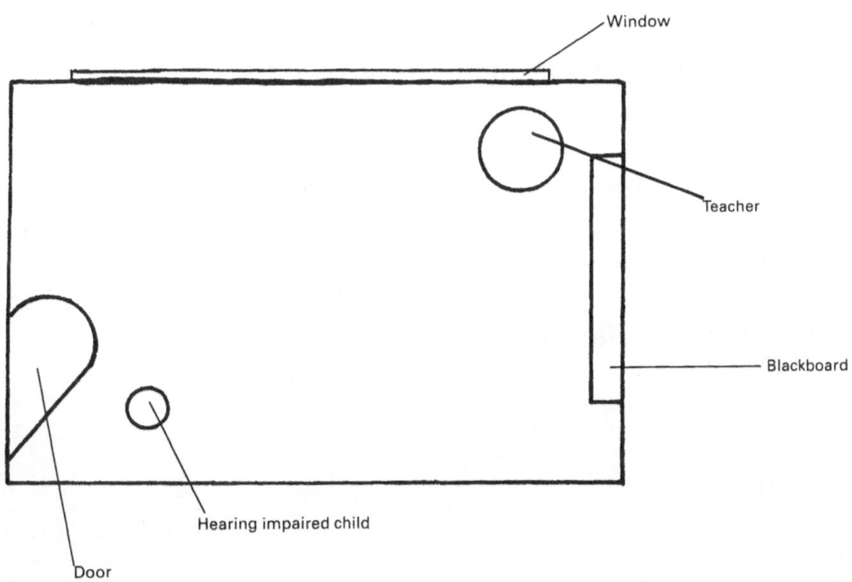

(b)

Figure 5.3 Seating positions in the classroom

(a) Good seating position: the hearing impaired child is seated near the front (good for listening and lipreading) and has a clear view of the blackboard. Light from the window falls on the teacher making lipreading easier.

(b) Poor seating position: the hearing impaired child is seated too far from the teacher and near to the door (noisy and distracting). Light from the window shines in the child's eyes making lipreading difficult.

- *Working with groups of children:* The group needs to be seated so that the deaf child can easily see the teacher and other members of the group. It should be a rule that only one child talks at a time and the teacher should ensure that the deaf child is aware of who is talking. Even within a small group it is helpful for children to learn the discipline of raising their hand when they have a contribution to make. If the deaf child is using a radio aid, other children in the group can get used to passing the microphone around.
- *Working with individual children:* This is an ideal opportunity to ensure the most favourable acoustic conditions (within the confines of a school environment). The deaf pupil should be sitting opposite the teacher or at least around the corner of the table to allow for ease of communication and also to give the teacher the opportunity to see easily any written contributions the child is making.

Summary

Schools are noisy environments. Noise levels and reverberation must be controlled in order to provide the deaf child with a favourable signal-to-noise ratio. Reducing noise levels should take place both inside and outside the classroom. Noise can be controlled at its source and absorbed by acoustic treatment. Amplification systems incorporating a short microphone distance effectively bring the teacher close to the pupil and thus provide a favourable signal-to-noise ratio.

Further reading

Berg, F. S. (1997) 'Optimum listening and learning environments', in McCracken, W. and Laiode-Kemp, S. (eds.) *Audiology in Education*. London: Whurr Publishers.

Flexer, C. (1999) *Facilitating Hearing and Listening in Young Children*, 2nd edn. San Diego: Singular Publishing Group.

Chapter 6

Systems in the Classroom

The problem in the classroom

Hearing aids work well when there is little or no background noise and the person speaking is close to the microphone of the hearing aid (no more than a metre away). In the classroom situation, the deaf child is rarely this close to the teacher and classroom conditions are frequently noisy and reverberant. Background noise is amplified by the hearing aid as well as the teacher's voice. If the hearing aid is turned up to hear the teacher when she moves away, the background noise will also be amplified more by the hearing aid. The further away the teacher moves, the lower the level of her voice reaching the child's ear and the more intrusive the background noise. Alternative forms of amplification have been produced in an attempt to overcome these problems.

Alternative forms of amplification

Radio hearing aids

Radio hearing aids, or personal FM (frequency modulated) systems are designed to overcome problems of distance and background noise. They are of great value where the child has to listen to one source of sound, for example to the teacher. Radio hearing aids effectively 'reduce' the distance between the source of the sound (the teacher) and the child, by separating the microphone from the hearing aid and placing it close to the teacher. The teacher's speech is then transmitted 'directly' to the child via radio waves. This has the effect of achieving a high signal-to-noise ratio.

There are two basic parts to the system, see Figure 6.1:

- The radio transmitter unit, which is worn by the teacher or parent (the person speaking). The microphone of the radio transmitter should be worn as close to the teacher's mouth as is practical; ideally it should be head-worn but more often it is worn on the chest. When positioned close to the mouth, speech into the microphone will be strong and clear. The signal is transmitted from the radio transmitter and is picked up by:
- The radio receiver unit, which is connected to the child's hearing aid(s). The teacher's voice is fed directly into the hearing aid from the radio

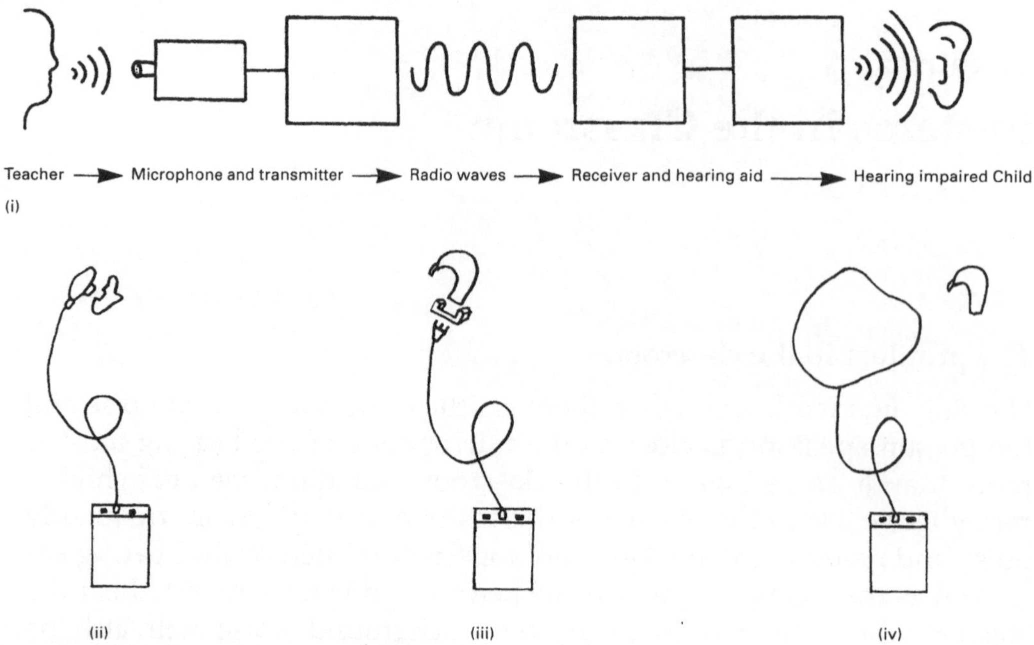

Figure 6.1 Radio aid hearing system
(i) the basic format
(ii) radio receiver and hearing aid all in one
(iii) radio receiver coupled to a post-aural hearing aid
(iv) radio receiver coupled to a neck loop, used with a post-aural hearing aid on 'T' setting (after Tate 1994)

receiver making it appear as if the teacher is talking close to the hearing aid microphone. The teacher's voice arrives strong and clear while the background noise remains relatively low.

A radio hearing aid generally works in conjunction with the child's own personal hearing aids. The addition of a radio hearing aid should not alter the signal received through the child's personal hearing aid (apart from making it appear closer and therefore louder and clearer).

It is important to realise that:

- the only feature distinguishing radio hearing aid systems from personal hearing aids is the favourable microphone placement
- the radio hearing aid is only as good as the personal hearing aid worn by the child.

Balancing

In order to ensure that the frequency response of the hearing aid is not altered by the addition of the radio system, the personal aid is 'balanced' with the radio aid. This is a simple procedure in which the frequency response of the personal hearing aid is measured and compared with the frequency response of the aid when connected to the radio system.

Since speech is presented close to the microphone of the radio, the signal appears stronger. The radio system is therefore tested using an equivalent, stronger, input signal. The gain is 'balanced' so that the frequency response is the same in both cases. Further details can be found in Appendix 3.

Radio aids are commonly used in mainstream classrooms. Therefore it is important that teachers of the deaf are familiar with the principles of radio hearing aids and their management and can explain these to mainstream teachers. This will avoid the situation in which mainstream teachers are handed the microphone at the beginning of a lesson and expected to use it efficiently with little or no previous experience or understanding.

Advantages and disadvantages of radio systems

- Radio aids pick up the sound of the teacher's voice and deliver it directly to the child's ear which is of great value in noisy conditions.
- In quiet conditions, where speech is close to the child, the system has no advantage.
- The radio aid must be turned off when not in use, or the child will continue to hear the teacher's conversation even when he is far away talking to other children – or even out of the room!
- It is important to realise that, when using a radio system, the child will not be able to appreciate the direction from which sound is coming.
- Although the child may hear the teacher clearly, he is not able to hear himself or fellow pupils clearly.
- The hearing aid may be equipped with an 'AM' (audio/microphone) switch to enable the microphone on the hearing aid in addition to the teacher's microphone. This will allow the child to hear sounds around him but this includes unwanted background noise and therefore is not always an advantage.

Sound field systems

A sound field system is a miniature public address system for the classroom. Sound field systems can help all children to hear more clearly whether or not they are hearing aid users. The improved level of sound in the classroom provided by a sound field system can be of particular benefit to children with attention and behaviour problems, to second language learners and to other special groups, as well as to children with slight hearing difficulty. Children who have temporary middle ear problems will find the system particularly beneficial.

The equipment consists of a microphone, amplifier and a number of loudspeakers, which are positioned at suitable points in the classroom.

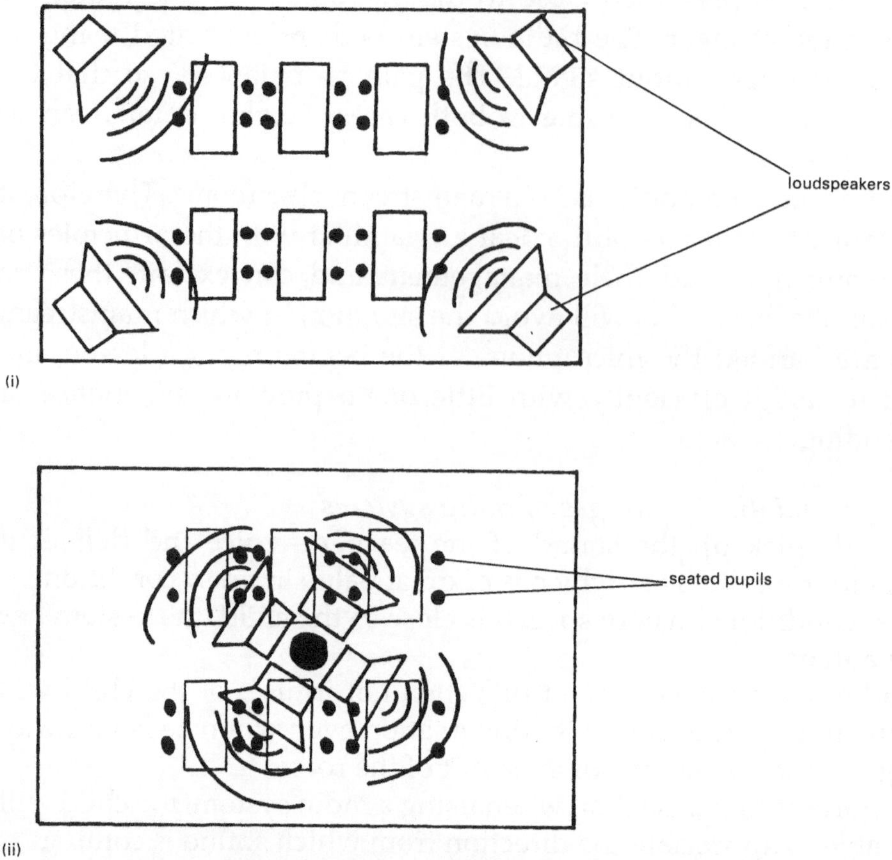

Figure 6.2 Sound field FM systems: Loudspeakers are placed, angled downwards, to provide an equal signal throughout the room
(i) Loudspeakers in the corners of the room
(ii) Loudspeakers centrally placed

The teacher's microphone can be wired into the system but the teacher has greater mobility if the system is FM. In this case, there is a radio microphone and transmitter for the teacher, exactly as in the case of a personal FM system. However, the pupils do not have to wear any equipment as the sound is delivered through loudspeakers. Figure 6.2 shows the basic parts of an FM sound field set up.

Loudspeakers are placed in the classroom in such a way that the sound radiates as evenly as possible to all the pupils in the room. Several loudspeakers will usually be needed to provide the required coverage for a classroom. Careful positioning of the loudspeakers is important. Sometimes loudspeakers are placed centrally on the ceiling in a cluster, each pointing downwards to face a different area of the room. Other placement possibilities include in the back corners of the room or on the walls, in each case high up, so that the sound path from the loudspeaker is not blocked by furniture or by children's bodies.

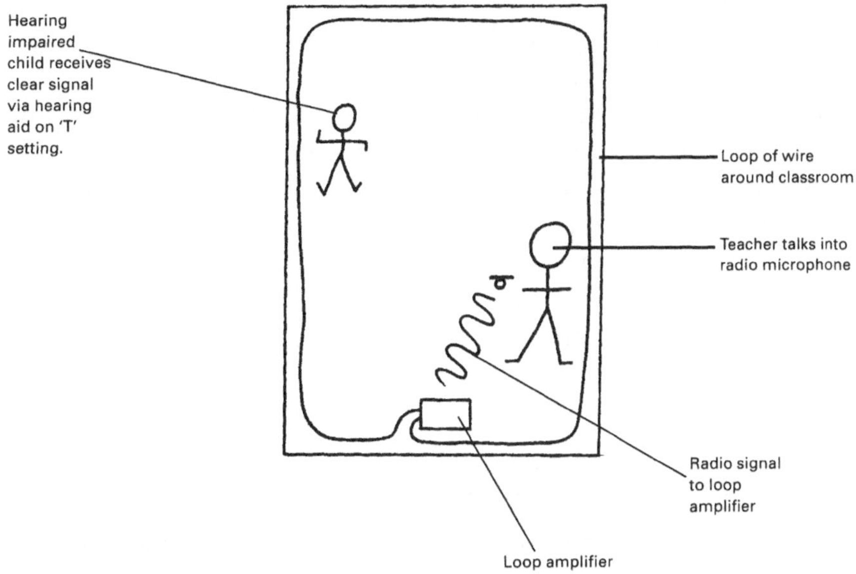

Figure 6.3 An induction loop arrangement

Induction loop systems

The 'loop' system (see Figure 6.3) overcomes the problems associated with background noise, reverberation and increasing distance from the sound source, in a similar way to radio hearing aid systems but uses magnetic induction rather than radio transmission. A loop of wire is fitted around the room and wired up to a microphone and amplifier. When switched on, a small electric current flows around the wire and this creates a magnetic field within the area of the loop.

A hearing aid equipped with a telecoil (switched to 'T', see Figure 6.4) will pick up the magnetic signal generated from the teacher speaking into the microphone. As the teacher speaks close to the microphone, a high signal-to-noise ratio is produced. The 'T' switch normally disables the microphone on the hearing aid. This means that background noise is

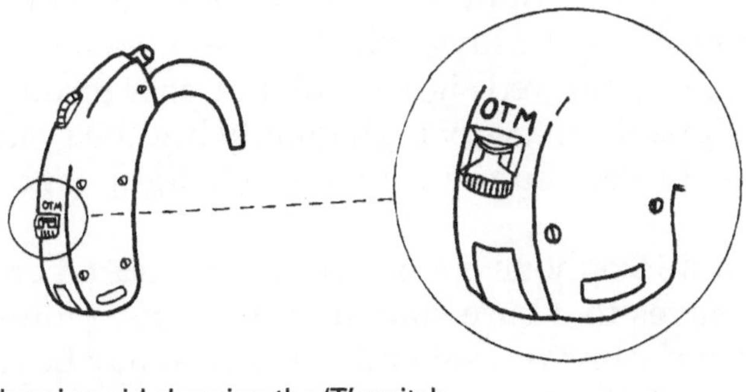

Figure 6.4 A hearing aid showing the 'T' switch
O = off
T= telecoil (loop)
M = microphone (on)

also cut out. If the child needs to hear sound from the environment as well as the teacher's voice, the aid must be provided with an MT (microphone and telecoil) switch.

A loop system is often used in public places, such as theatres and churches. When used in schools, the system is often provided as an individual 'neck loop' to be used in conjunction with a radio aid. A neck loop is a small induction loop, worn around the child's neck and plugged into the child's radio hearing aid. The teacher uses a radio transmitter. The radio signal is picked up by the child's radio receiver, which creates a fluctuating electrical signal around the loop and produces a magnetic field. A telecoil in the child's hearing aid picks up this signal without the necessity for a direct connection to the radio receiver.

There are a number of disadvantages to the loop system:

- There may be overspill causing interference if two loop systems are used in close proximity.
- There may be weak or dead spots within a loop system. With a neck loop, certain head movements may cause weak spots.
- Electrical interference from the mains, from fluorescent lights and from other electrical equipment, may cause strong internal noise in the hearing aid.
- The frequency response of the hearing aid set on 'T' may be different from the response on the 'M' setting. This especially affects the low frequency region. This may be important to profoundly deaf children as they may miss some of the low frequency signals on which they may rely.

The main advantage of a neck induction loop system over a radio hearing aid is cosmetic, in that the loop can be completely hidden.

Infrared systems

Infrared is another wireless option used in some school situations. Infrared rays are invisible light rays, which have a wavelength longer than normal light waves. Infrared signals will not pass through walls or other barriers. The signal is of a very high quality but the system cannot be used outdoors or in very sunny rooms as sunlight cancels out the infrared beam.

The teacher uses a microphone connected to an infrared emitter. This transmits infrared waves to a base station, or stations, mounted in the classroom. (Alternatively one or more microphones may be hard-wired directly into the system). The base station transmits the signal, which is picked up by infrared receivers worn by the pupils.

The major advantages of infrared signals over radio signals are that:

- They will not pass through walls or other barriers and therefore do not overspill to interfere with other infrared systems in adjoining classrooms.
- The signal produced is of a very high quality.

The major disadvantages of infrared signals over radio signals are that:

- They are adversely affected by sunlight.
- They do not work outside.

Auditory training units

Auditory training units, commonly called 'speech training units', are individual 'hard-wired' systems (see Figure 6.5). This means that the signal is distributed through direct electric wiring. The pupil takes off their own hearing aids and wears a headset, which is wired into the system. The microphones are also wired into the system. The unit may be powered by mains electricity or by a battery.

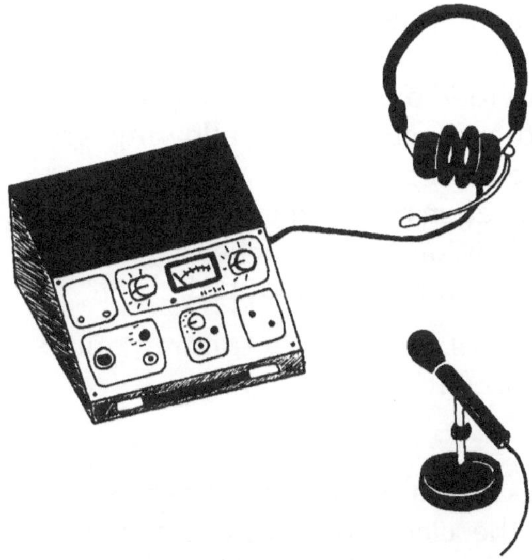

Figure 6.5 An auditory training unit

An auditory training unit overcomes the problems of background noise and provides the child, as well as the teacher, with a microphone close to the lips when speaking. The child can hear themselves clearly too, which is important for the child learning to monitor their own speech. There are individual controls for each ear. The use of headphones allows for increased output with minimal acoustic feedback.

It is important to ensure that the auditory training unit is set at a 'comfortable' listening level for the individual child. Children do not always select the best listening levels for themselves and the educational audiologist will ideally select the settings required for the child. Where this is not the case, the teacher may find approximate settings by comparing the dB levels provided by the unit and those provided by the child's personal hearing aids. A simple speech test may be helpful in verifying these settings. The unit should never be set so that it is uncomfortably loud for the child.

The larger components of the auditory training unit mean that it can provide a wider frequency response than personal hearing aids. This alteration in frequency response (a wider and stronger signal) is an advantage for those profoundly deaf children who receive a very degraded auditory signal through their personal hearing aids. However, it is known that consistent amplification simplifies the acoustic decoding task. Inconsistency means the child may hear the same sounds differently. This will make it more difficult for the child to recognise speech patterns. Children with less severe deafness who are good personal hearing aid users may be disadvantageously affected by changing the frequency response (Maltby 1999).

An auditory training unit has the following advantages:

- amplification is provided over a wide range of frequencies;
- sound is delivered via headphones allowing greater amplification without acoustic feedback;
- there is good amplification of the child's own voice (auditory feedback);
- there is good amplification of the teacher's voice;
- background noise is significantly reduced.

The main disadvantage of an auditory training unit is its large size and consequent limited portability.

Group hearing aids

A group hearing aid is basically a number of speech training units linked together for use in the classroom, where a group of pupils are all listening to one sound source. The system should provide each pupil with his own close microphone and be set to provide maximum benefit for each individual child's hearing loss.

Pupils remove their personal hearing aids and wear headsets, which are wired into the system. The teacher may use a wired-in microphone or, to allow greater mobility, may use a radio microphone. Each student has a desk or headset mounted (boom) microphone. The large size, with large components, allows improved quality and the system provides a good signal-to-noise ratio for the speech of the teacher and of each of the pupils. The problem of mobility is the main disadvantage. Group hearing aids are usually only found in special schools and units for deaf children.

Summary

Classroom conditions often produce a difficult listening environment. If deaf children are going to learn through audition the listening conditions must be improved. A number of hearing aid systems have been developed to overcome the problems of background noise and speaker distance.

Further reading

Berg, F. (1993) Chapter 5, 'Individual amplification systems' and Chapter 6, 'Sound field devices in classrooms', in *Acoustics and Sound Systems in Schools.* San Diego: Singular Publishing Group.

Chapter 7

Cochlear Implants

Introduction

> Paediatric implantation has been the subject of great controversy, but has also been described as the single most important development in the audiological management of deaf children in recent years . . . most teachers of the deaf, whether in the UK or elsewhere, can now expect to work with children using cochlear implants during their careers. It is therefore imperative that teachers in training and those seeking to update their professional expertise, should ensure they are aware of the issues concerning cochlear implantation. (Archbold 1994, p. 29).

Cochlear implants are an aid to the communication and listening skills of those profoundly deaf children and adults to whom conventional hearing aids offer only limited benefit. In most cases of sensori-neural hearing loss, the cochlea is damaged and the hair cells are not picking up the signals properly, so that the full message is not sent along the auditory nerve to the brain. Most mild, moderate and severe, and some profound, hearing losses can be helped with conventional hearing aids. However, it is now evident that the majority of profoundly deaf children will hear more with a cochlear implant than they will with hearing aids. Cochlear implants help by electrically stimulating the auditory nerve to produce a sensation of sound. As cochlear implant technology improves, it is likely that more children will benefit, and some centres world-wide are beginning to consider whether severely deaf people should be offered implants.

There are a small number of cases where deafness occurs beyond the cochlea. If the problem lies in the nerve or the brain, a cochlear implant will not help. An implant placed at the brainstem, further along the auditory pathway, may in rare cases be considered. There are also a few cases where the cochlea is very deformed or absent and it may then be that an implant cannot be used.

Cochlear implantion involves a surgical procedure in which an electrode array is implanted directly into the cochlea. The implant system includes a speech micro-processor which generates electrical impulses. These electrical impulses effectively by-pass the inner ear and directly stimulate the auditory nerve fibres (see Figure 7.1).

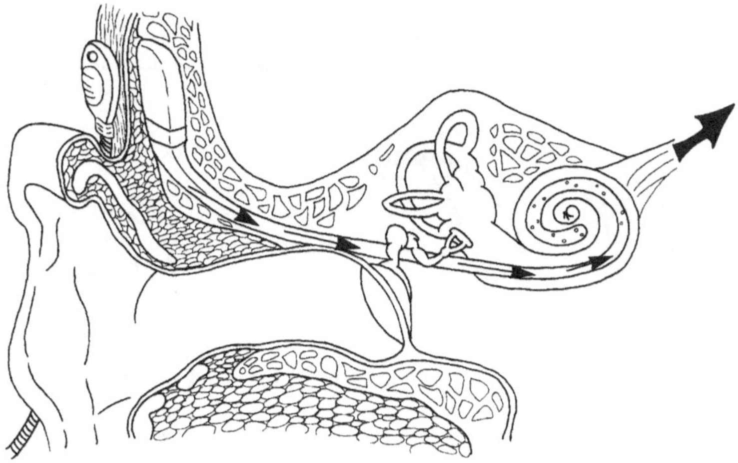

Figure 7.1 Electrical impulses travel up to the nerve of hearing (after an illustration kindly supplied by Advanced Bionics Ltd).

Components of a cochlear implant system

There are both external and internal parts to the system (see Figure 7.2).

External components of the system

The external components of the system consist of:

- The microphone, which is similar to that on a conventional hearing aid, collects sounds from the environment and converts them to electrical signals. It is worn at ear level. A lead transfers the electrical signal from the microphone to the sound processor.
- The transmitter rests on the skin just behind the ear and is held in place by a magnet. The transmitter transfers the signal from the external speech processor to the internal receiver usually by means of a radio link.

Internal components of the system

- The implanted receiver receives the signal from the transmitter. An implanted magnet attracts the external magnet and thus keeps the transmitter coil correctly aligned with the internal receiver. Some systems enable 'bi-directional telemetry'. In other words, there is an exchange of signals between the internal receiver and the external components, to verify that everything is working properly. An alert may sound/flash if it is not.
- The implanted electrode array (Figure 7.2) is inserted into the cochlea. Different cochlear implant systems use different arrays, with variation in the number and configuration of the electrodes, how they are positioned on the array, and the shape of the electrode array as a whole. Cochlear implant design is a highly sophisticated, rapidly changing field. It is important not to get caught up on minor details,

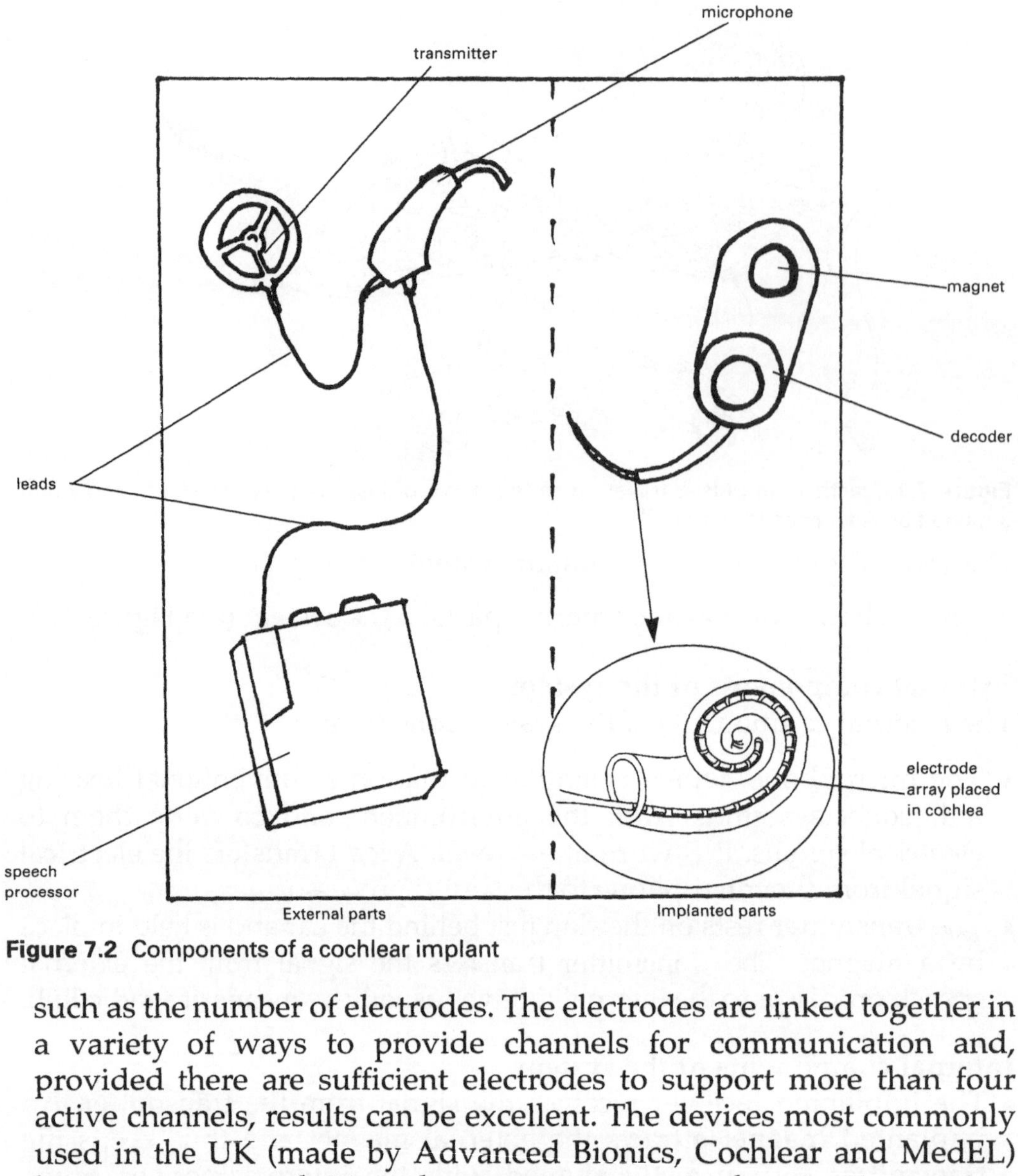

Figure 7.2 Components of a cochlear implant

such as the number of electrodes. The electrodes are linked together in a variety of ways to provide channels for communication and, provided there are sufficient electrodes to support more than four active channels, results can be excellent. The devices most commonly used in the UK (made by Advanced Bionics, Cochlear and MedEL) have given many children the opportunity to further develop spoken language through greatly improved access to auditory information.

The paediatric cochlear implant team

Children who have a cochlear implant are supported by a large multi-professional implant centre team, who work together with the locally based support team (see Table 7.1). The multi-professional team is based at and works from the implant clinic. The locally based support team works with the child at home and in school. In many cases, the roles of the implant centre team and the local support team overlap. For example, the teacher of the deaf from the implant team is likely to offer

The local support team (home and school)	**The implant centre team** (clinic)
Child	Child
Family/Other carers	Family/Other carers
Educational Audiologist	Administrator/Coordinator
ENT Consultant	Audiological Psychologist
Educational Psychologist	ENT Consultant Surgeon
Speech and Language Therapist	Medical Physicist
Teacher of the Deaf	Nursing staff
Other teachers	Radiologist
Other support workers	Speech and Language Therapist
	Teacher of the Deaf
	Other support workers

Table 7.1 The cochlear implant support teams

support in school and at home. Similarly the speech and language therapist and the audiologist from the implant centre will be interested in how the child is functioning with their implant in situations other than the clinic. Indeed, feedback from home and school is vital to ensure that the child's speech processor is 'mapped' correctly. The roles within the teams should be explained clearly to the parents and to the child. The child is the most important member of the team and should be appropriately informed about all aspects of the process, if of an age to understand.

Guidelines and criteria

Each implant centre has its own guidelines as to who may benefit from implantation. There are many similarities but the details may vary, for example one centre may specialise only in children under five whereas another might consider a wider age range. Guidelines are continually being revised in the light of new research; groups who were thought of as unsuitable for implantation a few years ago may now be considered suitable. Each implant team will have its own protocol for assessment. Most centres require that the child has worn appropriate hearing aids, with well-fitting earmoulds, for at least several months, and that they show little functional benefit from their aids. Aided audiograms (see Chapter 9) are often used to demonstrate lack of benefit.

At the start of 2000, children were being considered whose aided responses to sound field audiometry were worse than 55dBA at 2 and 4kHz. One function of the assessment is to ensure that there are no medical or radiological contra-indications to the operation. Children with difficulties additional to deafness were being considered by many, but not all, centres. Good educational support with a strong auditory-oral component, and a supportive, motivated family with appropriate expectations were both factors seen by many centres to be likely to affect long-term outcome. It was recognised that children born with a profound hearing loss, with little or no residual hearing, need to receive an implant early, during the critical period for learning language, so that early referral is vital to their success. In general, the age at implantation was decreasing, with many centres implanting children less than two years old. Some older children (over seven years) were being implanted, but these were generally:

- children who were born hearing and then became profoundly deaf following an accident or illness such as meningitis;
- children with a progressive hearing loss;
- occasionally, 'good hearing aid users' with spoken language skills, who were likely to do better with an implant.

While such guidelines are useful in providing a rule of thumb as to who might benefit, it has to be remembered that children are individuals, with their own particular set of needs and circumstances. Therefore all children should be individually assessed.

The stages of implantation

1. Evaluation, assessment and preparation for implantation

The child's ENT consultant usually makes the referral. Funding will then be requested from the health authority. The purpose of assessment is to ascertain whether the child will benefit significantly more from an implant than from hearing aids. Assessment generally focuses on:

- audiological and medical evaluations;
- language assessments;
- social, emotional and cognitive development of the child;
- support available at home and school.

During the preparation period, parents are kept fully informed so that, as well as realising the potential benefits of cochlear implantation, they also consider the limitations and possible complications. They need to appreciate the risks of surgery and to be realistic with regard to the long-term commitment required.

The child will also be helped to understand what is to happen and the implant centres provide simple booklets to help this process.

2. The operation and initial tuning in of the implant

Surgery time is usually two to three hours. A narrow line of hair is shaved around the site of the incision. The operation involves making a cut behind the ear and drilling space in the bone to accept the receiver. The electrode array is then fed into the cochlea and the skin flap is replaced and stitched. The child may stay in hospital for a few days.

The external parts of the system cannot be fitted until the wound has healed, which is usually about four weeks after the operation. The child will then return to the implant centre to receive the external parts of the system and for 'switch on'. The system has to be 'programmed' or tuned to suit the individual child. This is a gradual process and involves repeated visits to the implant centre over a period of time. The switch on (first tuning) session aims to set the electrodes at comfortable levels, neither too quiet nor too loud, for the child. The levels set are called a 'map' or programme. It may only be possible to tune a few electrodes at the first session. The child starts wearing the device, usually set at a conservative level. Over a long period of time, the child has to return for re-mapping to refine the settings used.

3. Management and habilitation

When the system is appropriately tuned, the process of habilitation can continue (it begins before implantation). The term 'habilitation' is generally used for children who have not yet learned spoken language, rather than 'rehabilitation', which is used for deafened adults or older children who are relearning their listening skills. Children who are implanted at a very young age may develop speech and language in the same way as a normal infant without active habilitation.

As with conventional hearing aids, it is expected that the child will wear the system during all waking hours. The child's family and teachers will need to learn how to check that the cochlear implant system is working properly, and to carry out these checks every day, as it must be maintained in good working order (see Chapter 8). The acoustic environment should be appropriate for active listening.

Initially the focus is on developing good listening skills. As Archbold (1997 p. 252) says, 'the major aim of cochlear implantation is to provide audition by which a child can acquire speech and language'. The benefits of implantation emerge gradually, over a number of years, as the child learns to recognise and use the sounds they hear.

The role of the teacher of the deaf

All teachers of the deaf are likely to be involved with deaf children who have cochlear implants. The situation and their role may vary depending upon their working environment.

- The implant clinic teacher of the deaf has a liaison role between clinic, family and school settings and is considered to be a key worker with the deaf child and their family. Teachers of the deaf working within the implant teams will be experienced teachers of the deaf with knowledge of various approaches to deaf children's language development, school settings and with experience of working alongside families of young deaf children. Their role in school includes:

(a) liaison with the teacher of the deaf, educational audiologist and other members of the local team,
(b) advising schools on appropriate listening conditions and activities designed to enhance listening and communication skills
(c) monitoring and evaluating the audiological, linguistic, social, psychological and educational outcomes.

- The local teacher of the deaf is likely to see the deaf child on a more regular basis than the teacher from the implant team and will therefore have a broader view of the child's needs. Much of the post-operative management will be the responsibility of the local teacher of the deaf. There should not be more support for children with implants than for other profoundly deaf children but the focus of habilitation may change following implantation. The local teacher of the deaf needs to work closely with the implant team to devise and implement strategies and activities for developing listening skills and promoting spoken language development, and to monitor and evaluate outcomes. They are in an ideal position to observe the ongoing use of the system and the child's everyday functioning with it. Their contribution to the initial and on-going assessment of the child is important.
- Peripatetic teachers of the deaf will have a role more focused upon advice and support to mainstream teachers who have children with implants in their classrooms. They may also be involved in visiting at home with the parents, although children who are implanted at an early age may need little in the way of habilitation, if tuned and managed appropriately.

Issues related to cochlear implants

There are many issues to be considered in relation to cochlear implantation. Cochlear implants benefit deaf children by giving them the sensation of 'hearing'. For this hearing to become meaningful and pleasurable requires a large and ongoing commitment on the part of the family and others working with the child. The habilitation programme, which is directed primarily towards developing listening skills and spoken language, is considered to be as important as the operation itself and without that commitment, the implant system will not be fully effective.

There are other issues surrounding implantation of which teachers need to be aware. It is not the intention here to provide answers or justification for a point of view but to highlight issues that teachers of the deaf may be expected to discuss with parents and other professionals.

The deaf community

Cochlear implants are generally portrayed in the media as a 'cure for deafness', a 'bionic ear', or at least as a means of minimising the effects of deafness. This suggests a 'medical model' for deafness where it is seen as a medical problem. Members of the deaf community, however, see themselves as members of a linguistic and cultural minority group. They do not see themselves as within a 'deficit hearing'/medical model, with a condition to be treated. From this viewpoint, to provide a cochlear implant for a deaf child is to affect a member of the community, and to threaten the community's identity and culture. Some members of the deaf community have likened cochlear implantation to cultural genocide, similar to that which occurs when children of other minority cultures are taken from their roots and brought up within a mainstream culture. They question the right of parents to choose major surgery for a condition which is not life threatening, with all its ongoing implications, involving a fundamental denial of the child's right to be deaf.

Expense of cochlear implants

Cochlear implantation is a very expensive and time-consuming procedure. Comparatively few deaf children receive cochlear implants. It is sometimes suggested that deaf children who have hearing aids are treated as the poor relations as they receive less input than cochlear implanted children. Where this occurs, the situation should be addressed, not by reducing the essential input given to children with implants, but by increasing that given to children with hearing aids. All children should have access to the best hearing aids for their hearing loss and to an appropriate amount of time and commitment to their habilitation.

Educational criteria for implantation

Criteria for implantation sometimes include a clause about the type of educational support the child will receive. It is suggested that support should include a 'strong auditory/aural component' (Archbold 1997, p. 245). It is important that children in educational programmes that support the acquisition of sign language as a first language and spoken language as a second language are not put at a disadvantage when selection for cochlear implantation is made. The children will need expert input to foster their developing spoken language skills, just as they do to develop their sign language skills. After implantation, deaf children have useful auditory information available to them and, although the implant team is not responsible for decisions regarding the mode of communication used, it is important that the local support 'team' adjust their communication to make effective use of audition.

Cochlear implants and sign language

Currently there is an assumption that once a child has had an implant then the subsequent support for language development and education should reflect the oral/aural approach.

The majority of children who may benefit from implantation are likely to be in the profoundly deaf category and may be already developing sign language as a first language. If the insertion of a cochlear implant will enhance spoken or written English skills, then it also has a place within sign bilingual education. Rehabilitation programmes devised for children with cochlear implants should rightly concentrate on developing spoken language. However, it may be argued that, rather than being a substitute for developing sign language, it should complement sign language. Deaf children, like other children, can grow up truly bilingual only if they receive expert input in both languages.

Summary

- Cochlear implants are an important development in the audiological management of profoundly deaf children.
- Part of the system is implanted but there are still external components to be managed and maintained.
- The surgery is but one part of the process; there also has to be a large and ongoing commitment to evaluation and habilitation, by all those involved – the child, the family and the professional team.
- A cochlear implant is another form of hearing aid and as such cannot restore hearing to normal.
- Any profoundly deaf child should receive a high level of support and there should be no more for children with implants. However, the focus of habilitation may change following implantation.
- Children implanted at an early age may need little habilitation.

Further reading

Archbold, S. (1997) 'Cochlear implants', in McCracken, W. and Laiode-Kemp S. (eds) *Audiology in Education*. London: Whurr Publishers.

Edwards, J. and Tyszkiewicz, E. (1999) 'Cochlear implants', in Stokes J. (ed.) *Hearing impaired Infants. Support in the First Eighteen Months*. London: Whurr Publishers.

Estabrooks, W. (1998) *Cochlear Implants for Kids*. Washington DC: Alexander Graham Bell Association for the Deaf.

Lane, H. (1993) *The Mask of Benevolence*. New York: Vintage Books.

McCormick, B. *et al.* (1994) *Cochlear Implants for Young Children*. London: Whurr Publishers.

Nevins, P. M. and Chute P. (1995) *Children with Cochlear Implants in Educational Settings*. San Diego: Singular Publishing Group.

Tye-Murray, N. (1992) *Cochlear Implants and Children: Handbook for Parents, Teachers and Speech and Hearing Professionals*. Washington DC: Alexander Graham Bell Association for the Deaf.

Chapter 8

Management and Maintenance of Hearing Aids

All hearing aids must be managed and maintained to obtain the best from them. They need to be free from feedback (whistling), distortion and unwanted noise. Simple daily checks should be carried out on all systems, with regular more detailed testing to ensure they are working well and up to specification. This chapter considers the maintenance of some of the common hearing aid systems. The guidance given here is of a general nature and much of what is written can be applied to other systems not specified in this chapter.

In all cases, the manufacturer's instructions must be read and noted.

Personal hearing aids

The principles of the different hearing aid systems are given in Chapter 4. The status and performance of a child's hearing aids must be checked daily and repair or replacement effected immediately if a problem is found. Children should receive a replacement of the same type of hearing aid, appropriately programmed or with the internal settings appropriately adjusted, if their own aid has to be sent away for repair. Daily checks are carried out by the teacher and by the parents. The aids should also be checked using a test box (an electronic hearing aid measurement system), as often as practicable.

The daily check consists of two parts: a visual check and a listening check. The following equipment (see Figure 8.1) is used in carrying out daily checks: stetoclip, puffer (also called an air blower) and new batteries.

Maintenance

The visual check

The visual check involves looking at all parts of the hearing aid for the following:

- cracks in the casing, tone hook, tubing and earmould;
- loose connections in the 'plumbing', that is the tone hook, tubing and earmould;
- dirt (including wax) or moisture in the microphone inlet, the tubing and the earmould;

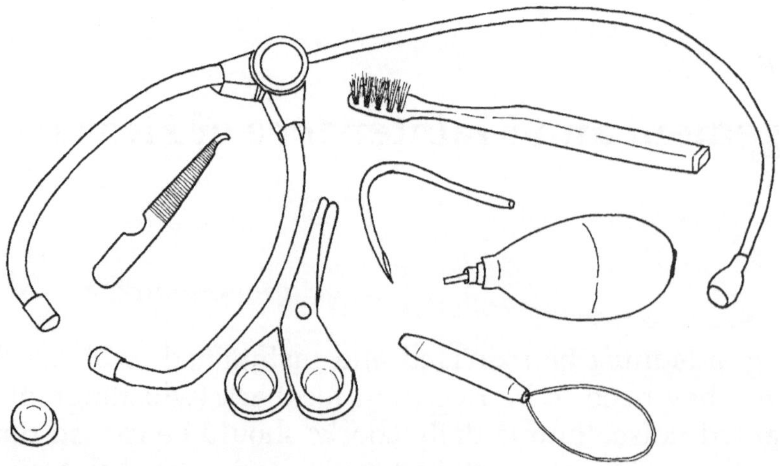

Figure 8.1 Equipment for daily checks (see Appendix 2)

- power supply faults, which are usually incorrect battery insertion or corroded battery contacts;
- body-worn hearing aid faults, which are usually damaged leads and cracked receivers.

Following visual inspection, the required action must be taken to rectify the fault.

Earmould faults

- The earmould can be separated from the hearing aid for cleaning. The hearing aid cannot be washed but the earmould can be washed with warm soapy water and scrubbed using a nailbrush or toothbrush. It must be thoroughly dry before replacing.
- Tubing can be pulled out of the earmould and replaced with new (see Figure 8.2).
- Moisture can be puffed out of the earmould, which must first be separated from the hearing aid.
- Most other faults will involve replacement of the mould.

Hearing aid faults

- A cracked or loose tone hook can be changed.
- Most other faults will involve repair of the aid by the manufacturer.

The listening check

The listening check usually involves a quick check of the battery, followed by a check for internal feedback and then listening through a stetoclip. At first the teacher will only be able to notice gross faults but, with practice, the ear becomes attuned and minor faults will also be noted.

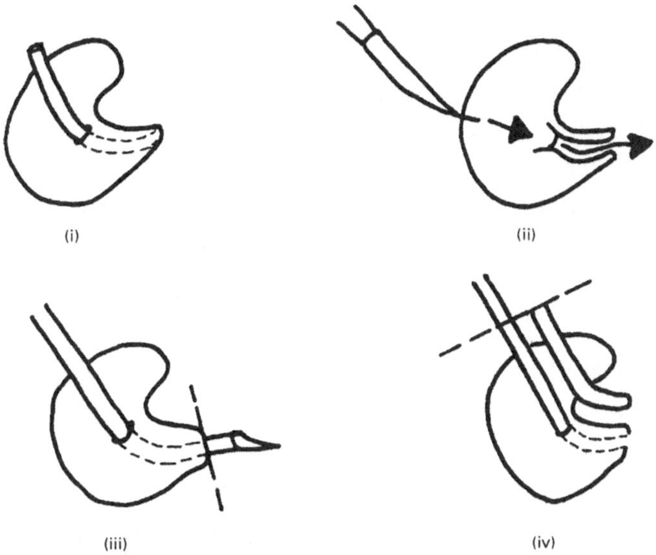

Figure 8.2 How to re-tube an earmould
(i) Remove the old tubing. Keep this for stage (iv)
(ii) Take a new piece of tubing of the same type and taper the end so that it can be threaded through the earmould
(iii) Pull the tapered point of the tubing right through the earmould. Cut the tube level with the mould
(iv) Cut the new tubing to the same length as the old one.

- *The battery:* If a battery tester is not available, the aid should be switched on and the volume wheel turned fully on. The aid is then cupped in the hand and a loud whistling sound (acoustic feedback) should be heard. If not, the battery should be changed. If the aid is still unusually quiet, check that the internal settings have not been altered. Batteries should be changed frequently so that they do not run out during the child's day. This is particularly important for young children.
- *Internal feedback:* Place a finger over the sound outlet from the tone hook. Feedback should cease, if it does not, tighten the tone hook and try again. Continued feedback points to 'internal feedback' within the hearing aid, and the hearing aid will have to be replaced.
- *External feedback:* The earmould should be re-attached to the hearing aid and a finger placed over the sound outlet hole in the earmould. Again, feedback should cease. If feedback continues there is probably a hole in the tubing, which should be replaced.
- *Listening through a stetoclip:* The aid should be listened to via a stetoclip (an earmould is not recommended because loud sounds could damage the listener's hearing). An appropriate damping filter should be attached to the stetoclip in order to protect the listener's hearing. The aid should be set at a comfortable level and listened to for the

following potential problems:
- no sound or weak sound;
- distorted sound, for example tinny or muffled;
- intermittent sound;
- added sound, for example hissing or buzzing;
- distortion or unusual noises when the switches or the volume wheel are operated;
- the leads of body-worn aids should be waggled to see if this causes any intermittency or distortion.

An example of a daily record sheet for checking hearing aids can be found in Appendix 2.

Radio hearing aids

The principles of radio systems are given in Chapter 6. Effective use depends upon management and maintenance. The following simple guidelines to use and care will help to ensure that the pupil gains full advantage from radio hearing aid use.

Management

It is important to be comfortable with the correct use of the particular radio hearing aid system employed. The instruction booklet should always be read and the controls fully mastered before the system is used in the classroom. Radio hearing aid systems are simple, but silly mistakes, such as switching off the receiver instead of the transmitter (easily done!), can render the whole system useless. The following points will help in ensuring the child receives the required signal.

- *Shoes and leads:* Ensure that the correct audio shoes and audio leads are used for the child's personal hearing aids. Audio shoes are available in many different sizes and shapes and some also have controls on the shoe. Euro leads all look the same but a few hearing aids need leads with different impedance.
- *Setting the volume control:* The radio hearing aid system should be 'balanced' for the child, by the audiologist or the teacher of the deaf. It may be helpful to mark the setting of the volume wheel on the receiver in some way, for example with a permanent felt tip marker.
- *Environmental microphone use:* Normally the child will need to listen to the teacher but will also wish to hear his own voice and to be aware of the verbal responses from other children within the classroom. Many radio hearing aids provide their own environmental microphones. Some radio hearing aids automatically disconnect the environmental microphones of the child's personal aids and use their own environmental microphones. This is acceptable but where this does not happen automatically it is

important to switch off one set of environmental microphones (either the radio aid or the personal aid). Having the microphones active on both the personal and the radio aids will cause excessive background noise to reach the child. Also the signals so received are likely to be out of phase (see Chapter 2), thus creating unnecessary distortion for the child. If the child is in a lecture type situation, it may be advantageous to cut out environmental noise by switching off all environmental microphones. The child will then not hear their own voice nor the children around but will hear only the teacher.

- *Transmitter use:* The teacher should use the transmitter to enhance the child's audition and should therefore ensure that the child is attending to the sound they are receiving. The teacher's transmitter should always be switched off when the child is not directly engaged with the teacher. If for instance the child is engaged in one mathematics task while the teacher is explaining a completely different mathematics task to another child, it is extremely unhelpful for the child to hear this. Information that is irrelevant to the child but picked up as the important signal by the radio will serve to disadvantage the child. This applies equally to the parent using a radio system in the home. When for example talking to the neighbour or doing anything in which the child is not an active participant, the radio transmitter should be switched off.
- *Battery charging:* Rechargeable batteries are commonly used in radio hearing aids. Recharging is a simple procedure but there are differences according to the system, for example in times required for charging. Batteries should therefore be charged according to the manufacturer's instructions.

Maintenance

A system must, of course, be in good working order and the teacher or parent using the system should complete simple daily routine checks to ensure this (see Appendix 3). These checks will include a visual and a listening check of each of the components of the system and of the whole system. The audiologist, or the teacher of the deaf, should make a similar check on a regular basis using a test box. The frequency of this check tends to depend upon the availability of the test box.

Daily checks

- The child's personal hearing aids should be checked as outlined earlier. The radio aid should be checked visually for signs of wear and tear, for example cracks, dirt, and worn leads or worn aerial.
- The radio receiver, with the radio facility switched off, should be checked as a conventional hearing aid. The battery condition can be assessed using a battery tester; alternatively, listening to acoustic feedback with the receiver volume turned full on will provide a rough guide.

- With a low volume setting, listen through a stetoclip. Talk into the microphone. Waggle the leads to listen for any intermittency. Move the controls to listen for crackling or any other problem. If possible, check at the level used by the child but NEVER cause yourself discomfort by listening at a volume that is too loud for you. A filter attached to the stetoclip will enable comfortable listening at higher volume settings.
- Place the transmitter near a sound source away from the receiver. Sometimes a colleague may speak into the transmitter for you, at other times another source, such as music from a radio, may be used. Ensure the transmitter and the receiver are both switched on (but not the environmental microphones) and listen to the quality of the signal through a stetoclip attached to the receiver.
- Turn the environmental microphone on and talk into this and listen to the sound quality.
- If the radio system is working correctly, attach the child's personal hearing aids to the receiver. Turn the environmental microphone off and listen through each of the child's aids in turn, via the stetoclip, to the distant sound source from the transmitter. Waggle the audio lead to check for intermittent faults.

Cochlear implants

Cochlear implants are hearing aids in which part of the device is implanted. The part of the aid that processes speech is worn externally. Like other hearing aids, cochlear implants need to be checked every day. Young children especially are not always good at reporting faults. The teacher of the deaf from the cochlear implant team should train the parents and the child's teacher so that they know how to check the system and what they can do to rectify faults. Trouble-shooting guides will be provided by the implant centre to help them.

A listening check is of no use for testing cochlear implants since part of the system is implanted; similarly the device cannot be run through a test box. Neither can another person with an implant listen to someone else's system, as the speech processor is 'mapped' or adjusted to suit the particular hearing loss. The speech processor would therefore be inappropriate, and may be uncomfortable, for another listener.

Visual check

An implant should be checked visually to ensure that it is switched on and that the volume and other controls are set according to the recommendations of the Implant Centre.

Most implants have a light, which flashes when sound is received. This shows that the sound is being passed from the transmitter to the processor. Talking into the microphone and watching how it flashes can test this. As with other hearing aids, familiarity with the correctly working system will help the teacher to pick up faults when they occur. Leads should also be waggled while the light is watched for intermittency. The sounds 'oo, ar, ee, s, sh, m' (often referred to as the Ling sounds) (Ling and Ling 1978) are sometimes used to represent sounds across the frequency range for speech. These sounds can be spoken into the microphone and the light should be seen to flash for each one. The child should also be seen to respond in some way. A child who has had their implant for some time should be able to detect each of these sounds at a reasonably quiet level and may be able to repeat them back. Most faults occur in the batteries or the leads. If there appears to be a fault, or if the child reacts unusually, each replaceable part of the system should be methodically checked and changed, using spare replaceable parts (leads, etc.) which should be kept at school and at home. If a problem persists, the Implant Centre and the child's parents must be contacted as quickly as possible.

The hearing aid test box

A hearing aid test box contains a very quiet chamber, the walls of which are padded with sound absorbent material. Basically the test box works as follows:

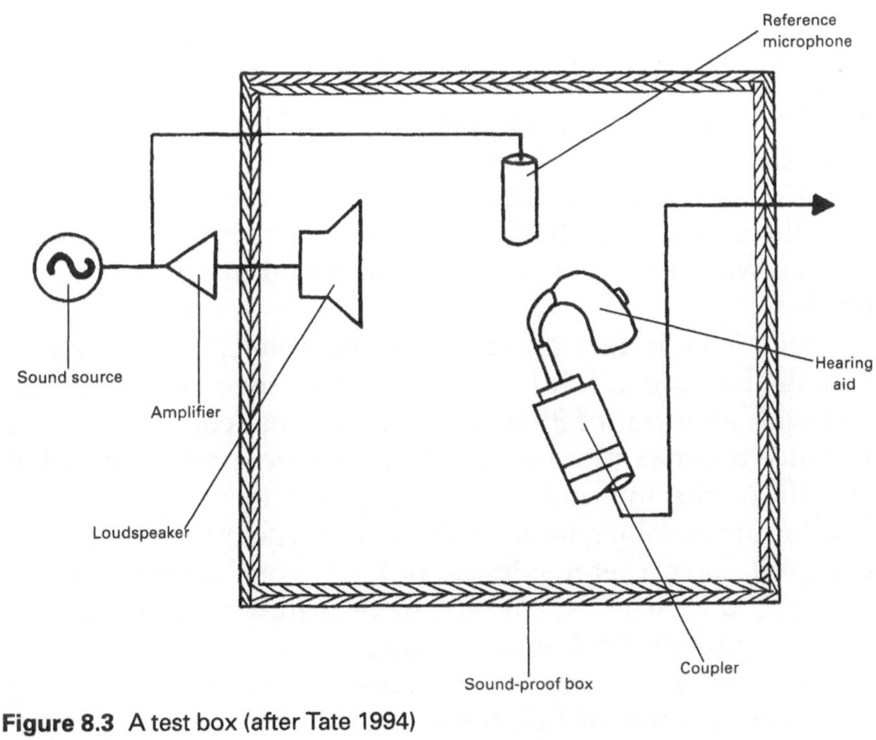

Figure 8.3 A test box (after Tate 1994)

- A test signal is fed into the test chamber through a loudspeaker.
- The hearing aid to be tested is placed in the test box.
- The hearing aid amplifies the test signal.
- The output (signal plus amplification) from the hearing aid is measured.

The conditions for measuring the output from the hearing aid must be standardised and accurate. The hearing aid test box components are shown in Figure 8.3. The hearing aid is placed at a specified point in the test chamber, this point is called the reference point. The sound in the test chamber is measured by a control microphone and maintained at the exact level required. The hearing aid is connected to an acoustic coupler in the test box. This coupler is made of metal and has a cavity within it of a specified shape and volume. The simplest type of acoustic coupler is the reference or 2cc coupler. This is the type of coupler that is generally used in test boxes. The coupler is linked to a calibrated microphone. The output from the microphone is therefore the output of the hearing aid under specified conditions. The output is recorded across the frequency range and this can be compared with the manufacturer's specifications.

In order that a hearing aid can be thoroughly checked using a test box (see Appendix 4), there are a number of standard tests carried out. These are set out in British and European (IEC) Standards, which ensure the hearing aid manufacturers carry out the same tests as the teacher or the audiologist.

Tests that are carried out most frequently to check children's hearing aids in school include the following: (BS6083: Part of 1984)

- *Gain:* This is the amount of amplification provided by the hearing aid. It is therefore the difference between the input and the output. The input signal used is usually 60dBSPL. If, for example, the input was 60dBSPL and the output from the hearing aid was 100dBSPL, the gain or amplification would be 40dB. (Gain is measured in dB, it does not have a suffix).
- *Maximum output:* This is the maximum sound intensity that can be produced by the hearing aid. It is measured with the volume control fully on and with an input of 90dBSPL. The internal controls may be altered to reduce the maximum output but the true maximum is that measured with all the internal controls also set to maximum. The output is the input plus the gain but this is only true up to maximum. A hearing aid will have a set maximum output above which it cannot go. For example, a hearing aid might have a maximum output of 120dBSPL, and a gain of 50dB. With an input of 90dBSPL the aid will still only produce an output of 120dBSPL, because this is its maximum. It is not capable of 140dBSPL.

- *Frequency response:* This is a measure of either the gain or the output across a range of frequencies. It is most usually presented as a graph.
- *Harmonic distortion:* All hearing aids add some distortion as a side effect to their amplification performance. Ideally the distortion produced should be much quieter than the signal going through the hearing aid, so that it does not cause a problem. Many types of distortion are produced but harmonic distortion is the type usually measured. Harmonic distortion is usually given as a percentage figure. The lower the percentage, the quieter is the distortion and the better for the listener. It is generally agreed that, for children, harmonic distortion should not be greater than 5 per cent. If a child is unhappy with their hearing aid and no other reason is immediately obvious, distortion levels should be checked as children can often detect small changes in distortion which are not obvious to the normal listener.
- *The child's settings:* Test box measurements are often made with the aid at the settings used by the child, rather than at the output levels set by the British Standards. If a record is kept of the output at these settings when the hearing aid is known to be working up to its specification, this can be used thereafter as a standard for comparison.

Summary

It is vitally important that hearing aids are always in optimal working order. For younger children it often falls to the teacher of the deaf to carry out routine checks, both visual and listening. Teachers should be able to do these quickly and accurately and have an immediate and appropriate back-up service for any faults found so that children are not without suitable aids for unnecessary periods of time. It is also important to encourage deaf children to become responsible for their own hearing aid maintenance and to discern for themselves when their aids are not working properly.

This chapter addresses: management and maintenance of personal hearing aids, management and maintenance of radio hearing aids, and management and maintenance of cochlear implants, and considers how these areas are related to roles and responsibilities of all who work with deaf children.

Further reading

Hodgson, W. R. (1997) 'Considerations and strategies for amplification for children who are hearing impaired' in Hull R. H. (ed.) *Aural Rehabilitation*, 3rd edn. San Diego: Singular Publishing Group.

Lewis, S. and Lyon, D. (1997) 'Management', in McCracken W. and Laoide-Kemp S. (eds) *Audiology in Education*. London: Whurr Publishers.

Chapter 9

Assessing the Benefits of Hearing Aids

Introduction

The audiologist prescribes hearing aids according to certain rules concerning the gain and output required for the particular hearing loss. The selection and fitting of a hearing aid is not an exact science and the benefit provided by the hearing aids must be evaluated. This can be particularly difficult in the case of young pre-verbal deaf children and a number of different tests may be employed. The principal tests are outlined in the following sections.

Tests used in the assessment of hearing aid benefit

Insertion gain

A hearing aid may be prescribed according to the amount of gain it is said to provide. However, every ear is different, and the size and shape of the ear affect the actual gain achieved when the hearing aid is worn. The reason for this difference is twofold:

- In large ear canals, sound from the hearing aid enters a large cavity and therefore the sound pressure level is weaker. In small ear canals, sound from the hearing aid enters a small cavity and therefore the sound pressure level is greater. For this reason, care has to be taken not to over-amplify the sound for children.
- The shape of the ear acts to amplify certain frequencies naturally, generally around 2–3kHz. Some ears have much greater natural amplification than others. When a hearing aid is placed on the ear much of this natural advantage is lost. The true gain provided by the hearing aid can only be found if the loss of natural amplification is taken into account.

Insertion gain (sometimes called real ear gain) involves recording the sound pressure level in the ear canal with and without the hearing aid. The difference between these two measurements is the insertion gain of the hearing aid.

The test is undertaken as follows. Test sounds are played through a loudspeaker placed a short distance in front of the listener. A small probe microphone, connected to the ear canal by a thin plastic tube, is used to measure the sound pressure level in the ear canal. The test is carried out first without the hearing aid and then repeated with the aid in place.

Insertion gain is an objective measure, it does not rely upon the child to respond. It indicates the gain available across the frequency range and is a useful measure in hearing aid fitting but it does not indicate how the child will respond.

Aided audiograms

Aided audiograms involve behavioural testing (see Chapter 3), and the child must respond to the test signal in a certain way. Aided audiometry is not objective and can be influenced by such things as tiredness and lack of concentration. The test results show the child's ability to detect tones.

The child's audiogram obtained unaided is compared with their audiogram obtained when using hearing aids. The difference between these two audiograms provides a measure of 'functional gain'. In order that a direct comparison can be made between the unaided and aided audiograms they must be obtained under the same 'sound field' conditions. Sound field, or free field, in practice means in an acoustically treated room, in which test sounds are presented through loudspeakers. These terms, 'sound field' and 'free field', may be used for any test given in such conditions, for example insertion gain and speech tests, as well as unaided and aided audiograms.

Pure tones are not used for testing in the sound field because the sound level is not standard but can vary considerably due to sound reflections, which cause increases and decreases in sound level whenever coinciding sound waves are directly in or out of phase (see Chapter 2). These increases and decreases in sound level are known as standing waves. To avoid creating standing waves it is common for the audiologist to use warble tones. These are tones that are made to warble (or deviate up and down in frequency) around the frequency to be tested. Sounds produced in the sound field will normally reach both ears and the test is therefore binaural unless steps are taken to block the ear not under test. If one ear has better hearing than the other, the binaural sound field test results can be said to relate to the better ear. Sound field tests must be undertaken in very quiet conditions as external noise can create errors in the results.

Aided audiograms are also sometimes used in schools to illustrate a child's aided hearing in comparison with normal hearing for speech sounds. The aided audiogram will therefore often show a 'speech banana' (see Chapter 2), as well as the child's aided threshold levels. By looking at which thresholds fall into or above the speech banana, it is possible to make a reasonable estimate of which sounds the child will be able to hear when using his hearing aid and which he will not. However, it is only an estimate because individual children can vary quite considerably in their ability to recognise speech sounds.

It should also be noted that hearing levels in dBHL refer to test results obtained under headphones. Hearing levels obtained in a sound field may therefore be shown using dBSPL or dBA (see Chapter 2). Estimation is made with the 'speech banana' shown on the aided audiogram (see Figure 9.1). Alternatively, the hearing levels may be converted to dBHL for direct comparison with the pure tone audiogram.

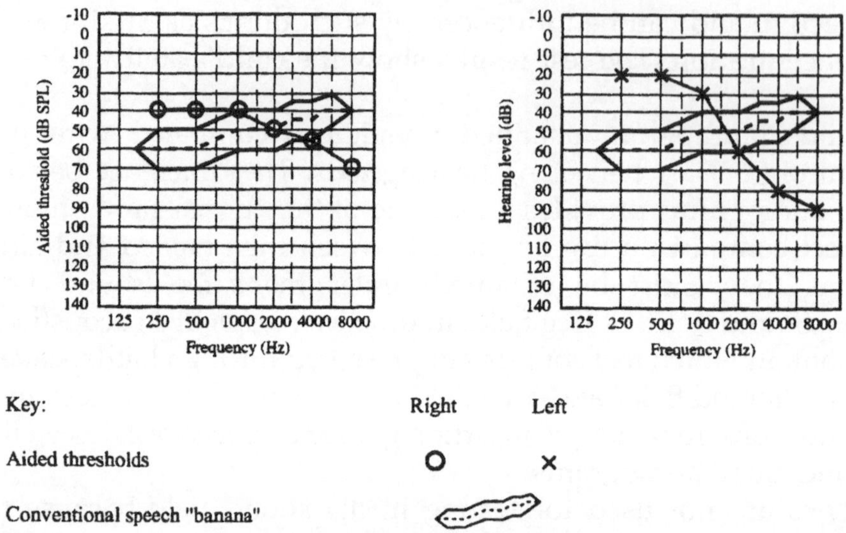

Figure 9.1 An example of an aided audiogram (diagram courtesy of A&M Hearing Ltd)

Speech audiometry

Speech audiometric tests are used to measure the child's ability to perceive and discriminate speech. Speech tests are of value as evaluative tests linked to the use of hearing aids. Speech perception is sometimes also used in diagnostic testing.

A number of different types of speech tests are available and there is a progression through the tests, related to age or ability and level of deafness. The range of speech tests include the following:

Toy discrimination tests (2 to 4 years)

Toy discrimination tests consist of selected familiar toys, which are set out in front of the child. The tester will say, for example, 'Show me the cow', and the child has to point to the required object. Young deaf children often do not have clear speech and an oral response is not therefore appropriate. Although toy tests are available in recorded form, they are often given using live voice rather than as a recorded version, because young children tend to respond better to live voice. When using live voice, it is very important to measure voice level and maintain it at a constant level throughout. There are a number of toy tests available, the most common are the Kendall Toy Test (Kendall, 1954) (Figure 9.2) and the McCormick Toy Test (McCormick 1977).

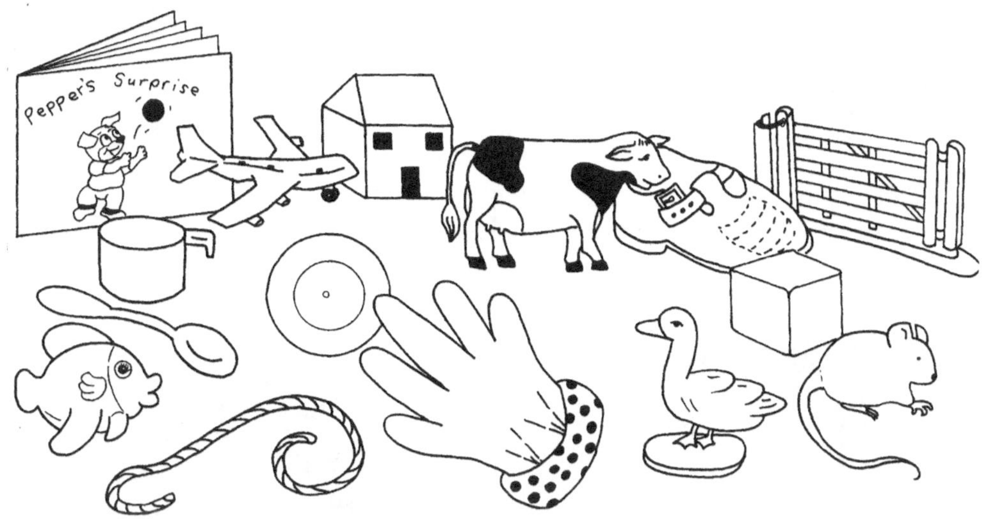

Figure 9.2 Toys for the Kendall Toy Test

Picture recognition tests (4 to 10 years)
Most children can attempt tests using pictorial representations, rather than toys, from about four years old. Pictures are presented in small sets. The child has to listen and then point to the word spoken. No oral response is required. A commonly used picture recognition test (Figure 9.3) is the Manchester Picture Test (Watson 1957), revised in 1984 (Hickson, 1986).

Word lists (8 years onwards)
Word lists usually require the child to repeat the word perceived and the response is scored appropriately. As a spoken response is required, poor quality speech may make the test difficult to score accurately. Single monosyllabic words, such as 'cot' are most commonly used. Some tests are scored by the number of words correct, while others, such as the Arthur Boothroyd (AB) Word Lists (Boothroyd 1968), are scored by the number of phonemes correct, for example 'f-i-sh' would be scored as three phonemes correct, rather than as one word. Lists are often presented in recorded form.

Sentence lists (8 years onwards)
Sentence tests allow for more sophisticated testing of speech perception in that sentences include the grammatical and semantic rules of speech, as well as the individual words. They therefore tend to test comprehension

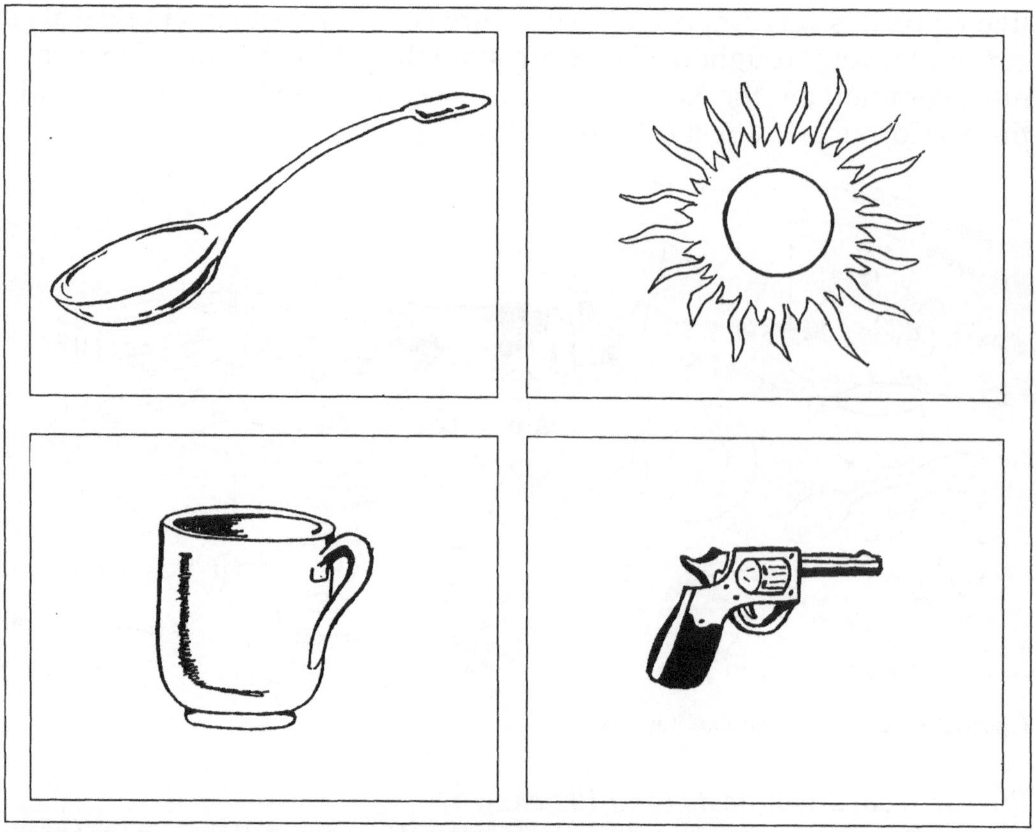

Figure 9.3 A page from the Manchester Picture Test (Hickson 1986)

as well as discrimination, which can be an advantage or disadvantage depending on the purpose for which the test is being used. Scoring is usually by counting the number of key words correct. The most commonly used sentence tests for children are probably the Bamford-Kowal-Bench (BKB) Sentence Lists (Bench *et al.*, 1979). The lists are available in recorded form.

Distinctive feature tests (for profoundly deaf children)

Profoundly deaf children hear amplified speech as a very degraded signal and will often fail to score on traditional speech perception tests. This does not mean that these children have no useful hearing for speech. Even minimal hearing can be valuable when combined with lipreading. The aim of distinctive feature speech tests is to measure the child's ability to receive aspects of speech perception which are important in distinguishing one word from another. The child is commonly provided with a choice and has to indicate which word was presented from a pair or set. The words of the pair are presented a number of times in random order to overcome the increased possibility of guessing. An example of this type of test is the Maltby Speech

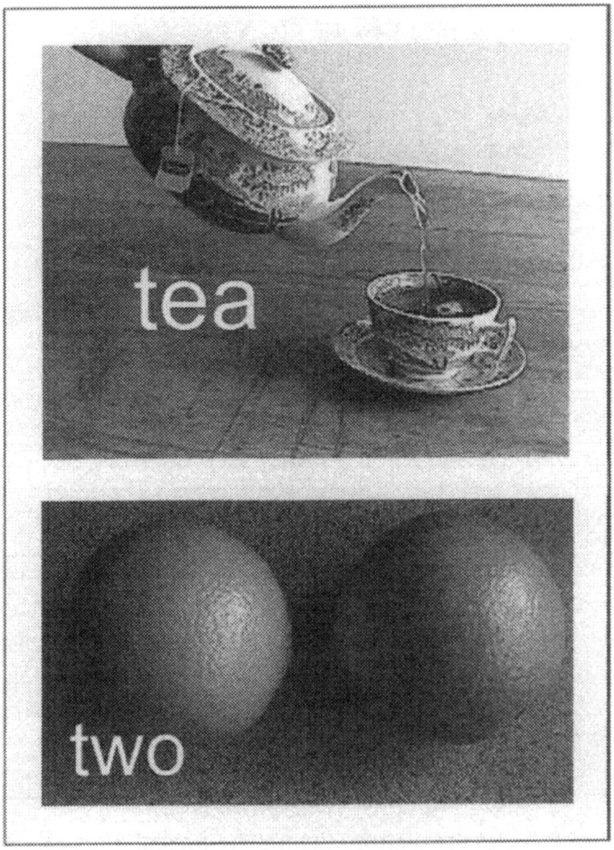

Figure 9.4 A page from the Maltby Speech Perception Test (Maltby 2000)

Perception Test (Maltby 2000) (see Figure 9.4). This test looks at cues to speech perception such as the vowel length, the number of syllables and voicing, and aspects of finer discrimination. It may be particularly useful to teachers (Maltby 2000b)as a tool for monitoring progress (see Figure 9.5) showing how well listening skills are developing over time, and indicating the effectiveness of hearing aids.

Summary

A child's hearing loss is individual to them in nature and degree, as is their ability to function with that loss. Hearing aids have a measure of adaptability and control over the level of amplification (gain) and output and the pattern of the frequency response. It is important that the gain and output of the hearing aids are matched as closely as possible to the auditory needs of the child. The most common ways of assessing the benefits of hearing aids include both objective and subjective tests.

- Insertion gain is an objective test, which indicates the pattern of gain from a particular hearing aid in a particular ear.

SPEECH PERCEPTION PROFILE:

Name ______________________

School______________________

100%											
90%											
80%											
70%											
60%											
50%											
40%											
30%											
20%											
10%											
	presence	on/offset	syllables	confusion	length	formant 1	formant 2	presence	voicing	manner	place
	VOWELS					CONSONANTS					

Age______ **Date**_________ **Tester**_________________

Figure 9.5 A child's speech perception from the Maltby Speech Perception Test (Maltby 2000)

- Aided audiograms are subjective tests, which, despite their limitations, give a clearer idea of the functioning of the particular child.
- Speech tests are subjective tests, which are used to test aspects of speech perception ability.

Further reading

Lewis, D. E. (1997) Chapter 9, 'Selection and assessment of classroom amplification', in McCracken, W. and Laoide-Kemp, S. *Audiology in Education*. London: Whurr Publishers.

Maltby, M. (2001) Chapter 4, 'Evaluation', in *Principles of Hearing Aid Audiology*, (2nd edn). London: Whurr Publishers.

Tye-Murray, N. (1998) Chapter 5, 'Assessing hearing and speech recognition', in *Foundations of Aural Rehabilitation*. San Diego: Singular Publishing Group.

Chapter 10

Teachers' Roles and Responsibilities

Audiological services

It is important for teachers of the deaf to be familiar with the audiological service with which hearing impaired children and their families will be involved. They are often asked to contribute to the information presented at clinic appointments and in some cases may accompany children and their families to the hospital. Their knowledge of how the child is managing their hearing aids and functioning in the learning situation will complement clinical testing.

The medical services are responsible for diagnosing deafness, prescribing hearing aids and monitoring the medical condition of the ears. Deafness is usually discovered in one of two ways. Some parents may suspect their child has a hearing loss and is not responding well to sound, for others deafness may be suspected at the routine screening test for hearing carried out by health visitors in the home or at the baby clinic. In either situation, the GP is the first port of call and if deafness is suspected the doctor will make a referral to the Ear Nose and Throat (ENT) surgeon at the local hospital.

At the hospital, further hearing tests will be carried out in the audiology clinic. This often requires several visits which, although frustrating for parents, allows for a battery of tests to be carried out by audiologists in order to diagnose the precise nature of the hearing loss. It is at this clinic that appropriate hearing aids are prescribed and fitted. The audiology clinic is responsible for the assessment and monitoring of hearing loss, and maintenance of hearing aids. Links with the audiology clinic and the ENT department of the hospital will be ongoing throughout a child's school days and beyond. This is necessary to ensure that appropriate hearing aids are always available and that the medical condition of the ears is carefully monitored.

A close link should be maintained between the audiology department and the educational services for deaf children. A teacher of the deaf is sometimes present at the audiology clinic when diagnosis is made. This allows for immediate contact to be made with the family and ensures that the teacher has full knowledge of the type of testing used and the diagnosis made. Many education authorities or schools for the deaf also have a qualified educational audiologist.

The educational audiologist

The educational audiologist is skilled in paediatric audiology, and takes a role that is distinct from but complementary to that of other clinical roles. This role includes collaboration with the hospital-based service to:

- diagnose hearing loss;
- prescribe and fit hearing aids;
- foster audition and maximise the use of residual hearing;
- advise on the provision of appropriate amplification equipment in school and home, including the use of radio aids and speech trainers;
- provide skills, information and training to other professionals and families;
- monitor hearing loss throughout childhood;
- refer conductive hearing problems to ENT departments for treatment;
- liaise with cochlear implant teams (see Chapter 7).

Cochlear implant teams are usually hospital based but include teachers of the deaf who are responsible for devising, implementing and supporting the rehabilitation programmes for children with cochlear implants.

The role of the teacher of the deaf

Supporting parents

Teachers and other professionals are currently encouraged to work with 'parents as partners' in all areas of education. From the Warnock Report in the late 1970s to the Code of Practice 1994, this issue has been highlighted and the role of parents has become more clearly defined and valued. 'It is important that parents and carers do not simply feel on the receiving end of advice, information and decisions, but are allowed to take a constructive role' (Webster and Webster 1997, p. 151).

There has been a long tradition in deaf education of 'early intervention' and working with families from the time of diagnosis of deafness. Early diagnosis of deafness and the introduction of appropriate amplification is widely considered to be of great importance in the acquisition of language (Watson 1998, McCormick 1993). Early intervention can be as early as a few weeks in high-risk babies and those who have failed a neo-natal screening test. Often, however, deafness is diagnosed in the second and third year of life. Support for families at this time usually falls to the educational audiologist, in terms of audiological management and ongoing assessment, and to the teacher of the deaf, who is the person linked more closely to family issues and the implications of having a deaf child.

Pre-school support

'The very first contacts a family has with support services, once a hearing loss has been suspected or diagnosed, are crucial in defining expectations, attitudes and confidence in what the future holds for a child' (Webster and Webster 1997, p. 345).

It is known that approximately 90 per cent of deaf children are born to hearing parents, who usually have little or no knowledge of deafness. Inevitably the reactions of most families to the news that they have a deaf baby are likely to be negative, emotional and very strong. Parents may be upset or devastated and are often aggressive. They may well be in a state of shock, which is followed by denial, grief, anger and guilt; symptoms likened to the bereavement process. These findings are widely accepted and are confirmed by Fletcher (1987), Marcshark (1997) and Moores and Meadows (1990). It should not be forgotten that the whole family is affected by the diagnosis of any specific need such as deafness, and this includes siblings, grandparents and all the extended family.

If support offered to families at this time is to be effective, it is vital that the needs of the family are identified.

- It appears firstly that the family needs time to allow an assimilation of the complex feelings and reactions that emerge. Parents need an appreciation from those supporting them that these feelings are common and natural, and that expression of them is totally acceptable.
- Parents need people to talk to. It is particularly useful at this time to meet those families who have experienced similar situations. Where it is possible to organise them, mutual support groups have been found to be of great value to both parents and their children. Such groups also provide an ideal environment for imparting and sharing information. Deaf people can discuss with the family their own life experiences and what it means to be deaf and, if it is appropriate, they can also introduce sign language.
- Parents need to acquire information. There is a wide variety of questions to be answered. Parents will need and want information about a whole range of subjects including the nature of deafness, educational placement, adult life and what it is like to be deaf. The support teacher of the deaf must be able to give information as and when it is requested. They must also ensure that, over a period of time, parents are made aware of all issues related to deafness and the implications of these for their child.
- Lorraine Fletcher (1987), who is the parent of a deaf child, comments upon the issue of 'information overload' and the balance between

wanting information and the ability to retain it. Parents like to have access to information as and when they want it and to be able to select appropriately according to their particular needs at the time.
- In the case of severely and profoundly deaf children, there are also immediate concerns to be addressed regarding the development of appropriate communication within the family. This question is of paramount importance. Teachers need to be well informed about the principles of early language development and about the variety of communication approaches and their implications for the family.

It is the responsibility of the teacher of the deaf (or the principle support worker with the family):

1. to introduce the family and the child to the variety of language approaches, including signed and spoken;
2. to guide the parents in developing an appropriate mode of communication with their child.

Deaf adults may play an important part in supporting hearing parents of a profoundly deaf child and can act as a role model, and as a linguistic model for the whole family, including grandparents. In this way, where appropriate, deaf children can experience both sign language and the spoken language of the home.

Gregory (1986) identifies with many of the needs of parents at this time and adds that whatever the parental reaction, most parents find themselves in a position where they are unsure and unclear about 'what to do'. Their primary need may well be summed up in simple terms – they need to know 'what to do'.

Audiological support

Audiological support to the family is of prime importance. Teachers must support the family in introducing hearing aids and establishing strategies for their use and management. Parents need to feel confident in the value and use of hearing aids, as the introduction of hearing aids to a young child is not automatically welcomed. Parents need to be shown techniques for checking and monitoring the use of hearing aids. A hearing aid checklist, which is useful both for parents and for teachers in mainstream schools, is given in Appendix 2.

Teachers of the deaf should be skilled in monitoring the language development of deaf children so that they will be able, in conjunction with speech and language therapists, to give appropriate advice and linguistic support to the family and to professionals in other social settings such as play groups. Where signed communication is used, deaf adults will also be involved in this way.

It is important that the nature of the relationship between parents and professionals is established through mutual respect. The specialist knowledge of the professionals and the intimate knowledge of the child by the parent should interact for the mutual benefit of the child and the family. Parents should be reassured that most of what they need to do is within normal parenting skills. Other new skills can be learned and absorbed into the parenting role (see also Chapter 11). It is important that the relevance of these new skills is discussed and negotiated with the parents. 'Any intervention should supplement and sustain the family's essential involvement in the child's learning' (Webster and Wood 1989, p. 29).

Statement of special educational need

The teacher of the deaf has a vital role to play in assessing the child's linguistic and educational needs and in discussing these with the parents. This will certainly include imparting information and also arranging visits to a variety of educational settings. The parents, and other professionals, will be involved in drawing up a 'statement of special educational need' which will suggest an appropriate educational placement and the type of additional support required.

Support in schools

Overall approximately 85 per cent of hearing impaired children are integrated into mainstream educational settings (Lynas *et al.*). The vast majority of these (70 per cent) are individually integrated into their local school and the others (15 per cent) are in units attached to mainstream schools or in resourced mainstream schools.

Support in the nursery setting

Where young hearing impaired children are placed in a nursery setting, it is important that it continues to address their individual linguistic and social needs while also providing access to the same nursery curriculum as their hearing peers.

As a very general rule, it is likely that children who are individually integrated into their local nursery will be those who are developing spoken language as a first language. Children who are developing sign language as a first language are generally placed in a mainstream or special school nursery with other sign language using deaf children.

Support from teachers of the deaf may be as a visiting/advisory teacher supporting individually integrated children or working with a group of several deaf children attending the same mainstream nursery. The role of the visiting teacher is to advise the mainstream teacher on a range of issues, including:

- appropriate activities for the hearing impaired child;
- strategies for communicating with the hearing impaired child;
- monitoring the child's progress and drawing up their Individual Education Plans (IEP);
- the statement of educational need and ongoing reviews;
- audiological aspects of support.

Mainstream teachers should be aware of the need to ensure an appropriate acoustic environment (see Chapter 5) and be competent in the management and maintenance of hearing aids (see Chapter 8).

Teachers of the deaf, working alongside the educational audiologist, may also be responsible for drawing up an Individual Audiological Plan (IAP). This monitors and targets the child's developing use of their residual hearing and their hearing aid management. It is an ongoing role of the teacher of the deaf, at all stages of education, to be involved in devising and implementing IEPs and IAPs.

Support in mainstream schools

For deaf children with a significant hearing loss but managing in their local school, support from a teacher of the deaf may be as little as a half-termly monitoring visit. This will be to discuss progress and problems that have arisen or are foreseen, and to ensure that mainstream teachers have sufficient audiological knowledge and skills to competently support the deaf child in their class.

Teachers of the deaf often become involved in providing in-service training to the staff of a mainstream school which has a hearing impaired pupil on their roll. This is the minimum entitlement for any pupil with a hearing loss. Further support may be viewed as being in response to a continuum of need.

In general, support in the early years of education is likely to be focused upon the continuing development of language, either signed or spoken. For sign language using children, English skills must also be developed for literacy and the subsequent access to the National Curriculum. The overall aim for deaf children is that they should become independent learners within the classroom and support should focus on appropriate linguistic support. Teachers of the deaf may be involved in support for deaf pupils for the national literacy strategy (NLS) and for the national numeracy strategy (NNS) (Charlton 1999).

The special school setting

Approximately 14 per cent of deaf children are educated in special schools. Many of these are now independent schools with residential facilities and take children from a wide geographical area. These schools are valued for the particular environment they offer, which includes, a variety of linguistic approaches, deaf-blind units and departments for children with complex needs. Most special schools establish links with their neighbouring mainstream schools to make integration programmes possible for some pupils.

Summary

This chapter has considered many of the practical aspects of the role of teachers of the deaf. They have a strong supportive role to the families of deaf children in the pre-school and early years. Not only should they be familiar with the practical aspects of support but also have an in-depth knowledge of all aspects of deafness. They must be confident in their knowledge as demand for information from parents must be responded to in a complete, balanced and confident way.

The specialist role of the teacher of the deaf depends upon their knowledge of the areas of audiology and language development in particular, and also of the learning styles of deaf children. If teachers of the deaf are well informed in these areas, their role in school and with the families they meet will be valued and respected. In summary:

- A familiarity with the audiological services, which are involved with deaf children, will enable the teacher of the deaf to support the family and offer informed opinions at clinics and meetings.
- Support to families depends upon the teacher's understanding of the implications of deafness for the family, thorough knowledge of all aspects of deafness and an understanding of the implications of deafness for child development.
- Support in school should be based upon an understanding of the linguistic and learning needs of the deaf child and viewed as a continuum allowing for individual children's needs to be identified and supported.
- Throughout the early years and school life, audiological support should be ongoing and consistent.

Further reading

Gregory, S. *et al.* (1998) *Issues in Deafness*. London: David Fulton Publishers.

Watson, L. *et al.* (1999) *Deaf and Hearing Impaired Pupils in Mainstream Schools*. London: David Fulton Publishers.

Knight, P. and Swanwick, R. (1999) *Care and Education of a Deaf Child*. Avon: Multilingual Matters.

Chapter 11

Developing Spoken Language

Introduction

Before children can be expected to develop spoken language they need to develop their attention and listening skills. For this reason teachers of the deaf need a knowledge of early language development, as well as amplification and acoustics, in order to encourage appropriate listening behaviour and to maximise the auditory potential of deaf children. This is important for all deaf children, regardless of their mode of communication.

Developing listening skills

'Hearing' is the reception of sound, whereas 'listening' implies paying specific attention to the sound, with the express intention of interpreting its meaning. The early skills required for the development of spoken language focus upon the enhancement of listening skills.

Early listening behaviour can be described as either reflexive or attentive. Reflexive behaviour is an automatic response to sound such as head turning (which is reflected in early distraction testing) or blinking. Attentive behaviour, in response to sound, has a more meaningful focus. Early indicators of attentive behaviour include smiling, eye widening, and an attempt to localise the source of sound. Observation of early responses to sound are important in identifying the auditory potential and listening behaviour of young deaf children (Carr 1997). These are particularly important for deaf children with complex needs.

Johnson *et al.* (1997) identified five developmental stages in the development of listening behaviour (auditory skills). These five stages involve:

1. Sound awareness; beginning to attend to sound; beginning to relate to sound as a meaningful event.
2. Beginning localisation; early sound recognition; beginning deliberate vocalisation.
3. Accurate localisation and tracking of sound.
4. Increased sound / speech comprehension; improved control of vocalisations as communication.
5. Early auditory comprehension; meaningful use of oral language; ability to initiate and maintain conversations.

A knowledge and understanding of these developmental stages on the part of teachers of the deaf and others supporting families of deaf children has a dual role. Firstly, it offers a clear structure to the type of support given to families of deaf children and secondly, it acts as a basis for assessing and developing a listening profile for young children.

Developing attention skills

Clear stages in the development of attention skills have been identified by several researchers (Carr 1997, Wood *et al.* 1986). These may be described as:

- *Disengaged:* Throughout the first year, children have little control over their own attention. Attention skills are fleeting and unpredictable and children of this age are highly distractible. Their attention shifts constantly to the most important and latest stimuli. This applies randomly to visual, auditory and tactile stimuli. At this stage it is important to reinforce fleeting attentions by touch or visual reinforcement and to encourage the child to 'see' sound as meaningful events.
- *Engaged/single channel:* Here the child begins to focus on one stimulus to the exclusion of others. For example, during interaction with an adult, the child may focus meaningfully on an object such as a toy and then on the adult, perhaps anticipating some reaction.

The child can focus their attention on a person and then back to a toy. It is clear that the child's attention has been 'engaged', but only on one thing at a time, and this is not yet the beginning of communicative skills such as turn-taking. Indeed the child's attention may wander between the object, the adult, and any other thing which attracts them. Gradually the ability to focus attention increases and the child is less easily distracted. However, they are still only able to channel their focus on one thing at a time and this is largely controlled by the adult or more sophisticated language user.

- *Dual-channel focus of attention:* The next stage is for children to have mastered the skill of attending to two things simultaneously. They may be handling a toy and vocalising at the same time, or listening to a sound stimulus while looking at a particular object. This skill may not be well developed and is still fleeting in many instances. This stage allows for the development of shared attention to an object, between the child and, for example, an adult. This shared attention to common objects or events is often referred to as the 'triangle of reference' and is considered to be an important stage in the development of the communicative process. If the adult and child are considering the same thing and one person is talking about it, then it is anticipated that the child will relate the spoken words to the object under joint attention.

Structured attention

Structured attention involves linking attention to spoken input (or vocalising) and attending to the object or event of interest. At this stage, the development of auditory skills through auditory training becomes a realistic option.

Auditory training should permeate everyday life as well as involving a planned teaching programme carried out at a certain time and place. To maximise benefit from auditory training, these two components must be linked and mutually supportive.

Facilitating language development

Providing an environment that is rich in natural, meaningful interactions best facilitate language development. The home environment is a rich and stimulating auditory environment (sometimes called a 'soundscape'), where children's language develops fully during the course of normal parenting and family life.

Most parents are natural and skilled 'teachers' of language to their own children. Therefore support should enable and encourage parents to realise and use the skills they already have, in a natural and confident way that is appropriate to a deaf child.

The following aspects of communication, used by parents of young children, have been identified as particularly supportive to language development:

- Short simple sentences, which are contingent upon the current circumstances.
- A higher register of voice with a strong rhythm and intonation pattern presented. The term used for this type of language is 'Motherese' or 'child directed speech'. This second term reflects our understanding of the child as an equal partner in the communicative process where adults tend to adapt their language style according to the response they get from the child.
- Utterances from the child that are extended and clarified.

It is often helpful for parents to identify certain periods of 'quality auditory time' in the day, when competing noise is at a minimum and when activities can be focused on appropriate games and activities to further enhance the child's listening skills. Parents should be encouraged to share household and play activities with their children and to play turn-taking games. This type of activity provides the sort of input required for language development. Finger games, singing games and nursery rhymes are all a rich source of linguistic input offering rhythm, intonation and repetition. There are many published programmes and ideas for developing listening skills. What is common to all programmes is that:

- the activities are fun for the children
- they incorporate everyday toys and objects within the home
- they link closely to the sort of interactions or games that parents and carers play with their children anyway.

The principles of auditory training relate equally to developing spoken language in children who have had cochlear implants and in those who are more conventionally aided.

The role of the teacher of the deaf

The parent–teacher partnership

It is important that the parent–teacher relationship is seen as a partnership of equals. The role of the teacher is one of assessing the skills and needs of the individual family and planning a programme of support to reflect those needs, with ideas and strategies for developing residual hearing imparted to the family as and when appropriate.

Some parents like to have a specific programme developed for them to work through as they then feel reassured that they are doing all 'the right things'. Others find that kind of formal working difficult and any suggestion that they have to become 'teacher' to their child is threatening. Because teachers of the deaf are skilled and experienced, they can appear more successful than parents in communicating with deaf children. In this situation it is likely that parents may feel vulnerable and de-skilled. The teacher of the deaf should therefore:

- see each family as an individual unit with their own specific needs;
- be sensitive to the differing skills and confidence of each family;
- develop realistic and appropriate programmes of support;
- work in close partnership with parents.

The use of hearing aids

Parents should be encouraged to provide a sympathetic acoustic environment in the home, particularly when young children are being introduced to hearing aids. The acoustic advantages of curtains and carpets and soft furnishings should be maximised (see Chapter 5) and conflicting and competing noise should be minimised. This includes simple things like turning the television or radio off when talking to the child.

Every support and encouragement should be given to parents in establishing a positive hearing aid regime. In general, parents should be encouraged to:

- be relaxed but firm about hearing aids;
- distract the child's attention from the aids;
- reward success.

It is important is that parents should not view themselves as 'failures' or their children as difficult because of a lack of success early on. A good working partnership between the parents and the teacher of the deaf should provide the parents with the necessary continuing support and encouragement.

Assessment

An important part of the teacher of the deaf's role is assessing the developing skills of the child both in the areas of:

- hearing aid wearing and management, and
- developing listening and language skills.

It is important that teachers find an easy, accessible and non-threatening method of recording assessment. Developing profiles and portfolios are appropriate ways of doing this and of course parents can contribute to and indeed keep these records and assessments at home. Parents have a vital role in assessment as they know their own child best and are generally acute and accurate observers of them. With parents' help, targets for both language development and hearing aid wearing can be produced from the profiles of development. It can be very encouraging for parents to be able to note and record even small steps of progress. Targets can be recorded in the form of a 'family plan' or an individual learning programme, which can give a realistic, but manageable, structure to the support given to the parents, with clear indications about how to proceed.

Assessment of the auditory potential and linguistic progress of individual children is crucial in planning for their future educational placement and the type of support they will need in school. The teacher of the deaf has a vital role in contributing to the drawing up of statements of special educational need.

The role of the speech and language therapist

Speech and language therapists are an invaluable part of the inter-disciplinary team working with deaf children. They work closely with teachers of the deaf and other involved professionals, sharing skills and information. Their primary role is to assess and develop language and they need to understand child development in its fullest sense. The speech and language therapist will assess the developing language of the child and devise appropriate programmes of work which may be introduced in the clinic, but with the intention of the approach and work continuing in the home and/or nursery or school. Some speech and language therapists are based in schools and nurseries where they are able to work with children in their usual setting, as well as working alongside teachers and nursery nurses. Some speech and language therapists work with deaf children as part of their generic role, but many have chosen to specialise in this area.

Much of the speech and language therapist's time is spent working with individual children. Clearly, for the purposes of assessment and introducing new programmes, working in a one-to-one situation with children is ideal. Many speech and language therapists also like to involve children and their families in group sessions. Group games and activities and conversations can be used to establish turn-taking and other language skills. Groups have the advantages that:

- there is less individual pressure on the child to 'perform';
- there is opportunity for children to have reinforcement by watching and listening to others;
- it is easier to produce a natural linguistic environment;
- the group environment may be more relaxed and more fun.

The speech and language therapist will diagnose the precise nature of a deaf child's linguistic difficulties and differentiate between those problems caused directly by hearing loss and those associated with other specific language difficulties. Deaf children will experience specific language difficulties in the same proportion as hearing children, so it is likely that the teacher of the deaf will meet some deaf children who have an additional language problem.

It is vital that there is a good communication between parents, teachers of the deaf, speech and language therapists and all other involved professionals. Clear and accessible records need to be kept of meetings and information so that support is consistent from all involved people.

Summary

The auditory skills and spoken language of all deaf children should be developed to their fullest potential. This can be viewed as the child's right and is an inherent part of the role of the teacher of the deaf. The speech and language therapist works with teachers of the deaf to assess and develop the child's linguistic skills, and to enable parents to assume their natural role within this process.

When developing spoken communication, it is important that:

- the child is attending visually and/or auditorily;
- the language used is clear and simple;
- the language used is meaningful to the context;
- there is turn-taking during the communication;
- parents respond to and extend the child's language;
- parents share enjoyable auditory activities, such as singing games, nursery rhymes and finger rhymes with their children.

All parents have natural skills to help develop their children's language. Deafness may interrupt the process and parents therefore need support to establish good quality natural communication.

Further reading

Archbold, S. and Tait, M. (1994) 'Rehabilitation – a practical approach', in McCormick B. *et al.* (eds) *Cochlear implants for young children.* London: Whurr Publishers.

Carr, G. (1997) 'Development of listening skills', in McCracken, W. and Laoide-Kemp, S. (eds) *Audiology in Education.* London: Whurr Publishers.

Dyar, D. (1994) 'Monitoring progress – the role of the speech and language therapist', in McCormick, B. *et al.* (eds) *Cochlear Implants for Young Children,* London:Whurr.

Flexer, C. (1994) *Facilitating hearing and listening in young children.* San Diego: Singular Publishing Group.

Webster, V. and Webster, A. (1997) 'Raising achievement in hearing impaired pupils', in *Support Matters 14–15.* Bristol: Avec Designs Ltd.

Appendix 1

Audiological descriptors (British Association of Teachers of the Deaf 1981, amended 1985)

The National Executive Council (NEC) has agreed on descriptors for the following audiological terms:

Average hearing loss
Prelingual hearing loss
Slightly hearing-impaired
Moderately hearing-impaired
Severely hearing-impaired
Profoundly hearing-impaired.

Methods of calculation

The average hearing loss of a child should be calculated in the following way. The loss in dB (HL) at the five frequencies 250Hz, 500Hz, 1 kHz, 2kHz and 4kHz should be averaged for each ear. The ear which shows the smaller loss (i.e. the better ear) is then taken as the child's *average hearing loss*.

If there is no response at any of the five frequencies, then, for the purposes of the calculation, a numerical value is given to that no response (NR). The numerical value given is 130 dBHL.

e.g.

Frequency	250Hz	500Hz	1kHz	2kHz	4kHz
Left ear	80	90	100	NR	110
Right ear	60	80	90	110	NR

The average loss in the left ear is:

$$\frac{80+90+100+130+110}{5} = \frac{510}{5} = 102 \text{ dBHL}$$

The average loss in the right ear is:

$$\frac{60+80+90+110+130}{5} = \frac{470}{5} = 94 \text{ dBHL}$$

The average hearing loss is 94 dBHL.

Descriptors

- Average hearing loss: the average of five frequencies (250 – 4kHz).
- Prelingual loss: onset before the age of 18 months.
- Slightly hearing-impaired: children whose average loss does not exceed 40 dBHL.
- Moderately hearing-impaired: children whose average loss is from 41–70 dBHL.
- Severely hearing-impaired: children whose average loss is from 71–95dBHL.
- Profoundly hearing-impaired: children whose average loss exceeds 95 dBHL.

Appendix 2

Checking hearing aids

Recording hearing aid information

All teachers should keep a record of hearing aids used by their pupils and the prescribed settings. The type of information needed for each hearing aid includes:

Child's name		
Make of aid		
Model		
Serial number		
Internal settings		
Battery type		
Volume setting		
Hook/elbow		
(BW) Receiver number		

Equipment

A teacher with a hearing-aided pupil in the class should have the following equipment available for daily checks and repairs:

- Stetoclip (with filter as necessary) for listening to hearing aids.
- Toothbrush or nail brush for cleaning dirty earmoulds. Earmoulds should be detached from the hearing aids and washed in warm soapy water. They must be dried thoroughly before re-attaching.
- Puffer to blow out moisture from earmould and tubing.
- Nail file to smooth rough edges on earmoulds.

- Pre-bent tubing for replacing old or damaged tubing.
- Thin wire or a re-tubing tool for pulling tubing through earmould.
- Scissors for cutting tubing.
- Batteries for replacement as necessary.

Simple daily hearing aid checks

Visual checks

1. Look at the earmould for:
   - dirt and wax;
   - splits or cracks;
   - rough edges.
2. Look at the aid for:
   - cracks in the aid / elbow;
   - loose connections in the 'plumbing' (elbow, tubing and earmould);
   - corroded battery contacts;
   - battery placed incorrectly.

Listening checks

1. Switch the aid on. Turn the volume full on. Cup your hand around the hearing aid. It should whistle (feedback) loudly. (If there is no whistling, check the battery and also ensure the sound outlet is not blocked).
2. Place your finger over the sound outlet on the earmould. The whistling should cease. (If not, check the earmould).
3. Detach the earmould from the aid. Place your finger over the end of the elbow of the hearing aid. The whistling should cease. (If not, check the elbow for cracks or replace the hearing aid).
4. Listen to the aid using the stetoclip. (High sound levels may damage your hearing. Use only at low volume or attach an appropriate filter).

Using a stetoclip

1. Turn the aid's volume to minimum and switch the aid off.
2. Disconnect the earmould from the aid.
3. Connect the stetoclip to the hearing aid elbow.
4. Switch the aid on and slowly increase the volume until it is at a comfortable level for you.
5. Talk into the aid. You could say a couple of lines of a nursery rhyme or count up to ten. You might then say sounds to test listening for low and high frequencies, for example:
   'go go sh sh' or 'ee oo ar mm s sh'
6. You should:
   - ensure the aid is working;
   - note any changes in the quality or loudness of the aid (if you notice a problem, try a new battery and then listen again);
   - move the switches (and leads if the aid is body-worn) and listen for distortion, buzzing, hissing, crackling or intermittency.

Appendix 3

Checking radio hearing aids

Radio aids are not difficult to test but require the teacher to ensure each part is working separately as well as together. The manufacturer's instructions should always be read before first use. The following are general guidelines:

1. The child's personal hearing aids must be checked as set out in the previous sections.
2. Check the radio aid visually for signs of damage.
3. When the radio transmitter and receiver are switched on, the battery light on each should glow momentarily.
4. Give the transmitter to another person and ask them to talk into it. Alternatively place the transmitter near to a stereo or other sound source. Check the radio aid by listening through the receiver using a stetoclip. Listen for smooth clear sound. (If there is a problem, make sure the transmitter and receiver are switched on. If there is still a problem, try changing the microphone and if necessary the aerial. If this does not solve the problem, you will need to use another transmitter.)
5. Attach the hearing aids to the radio receiver and listen to the whole system. Wiggle the leads and listen for any intermittency or distortion of the signal. (If there is a problem, change the leads and if necessary the connecting 'shoes'.)

Teachers of the deaf will check/balance radio aids also using a test box. Again, this is not a difficult procedure. The idea of checking a radio aid in a test box is to ensure no change is made to the overall frequency response of the hearing aids by adding the radio receiver/transmitter. The test is performed as follows:

- The transmitter is placed in the test box.
- The receiver and the hearing aid, attached to the coupler, are all placed outside the test box.
- The input signal is increased to 75dBSPL to take account of the increased input when the teacher speaks close to the microphone of the transmitter.
- An output frequency response curve is recorded.
- The frequency response is compared to that obtained from the hearing aid alone (see earlier) and adjusted to match as closely as possible. The printout can be retained for future comparison.

Appendix 4

General instructions for use of a test box

Checks using a test box should be made at regular intervals. Audiologists will use a test box to check that hearing aids are working to specification according to British Standard tests. Teachers are more likely to be interested in the performance of the child's aids as they are usually used. For this purpose, a note should be kept of the internal settings and the volume control level used and the teacher should print out and keep an output frequency response curve for each aid. This should be done when the aids are new. These frequency response curves can be used as a baseline for comparison thereafter.

Test boxes are not identical and the manufacturer's instructions should always be read before first use.

Calibration

1. Switch the machine on.
2. Place the microphone in the soundproof chamber. There should be a marking, such as a white dot, to indicate the exact position of the microphone. The microphone should be placed facing the sound inlet grille.
3. Press 'level'. You will hear the machine running through the frequencies as it calibrates itself.
4. Check the calibration. Make adjustment if necessary. The box must be re-calibrated after any adjustment has been made.

Using the test box to carry out a quick hearing aid test at user volume and settings

1. Check the hearing aid visually and check for acoustic feedback. (Replace the battery if necessary.)
2. Turn the aid to user volume and switch on.
3. Connect the hearing aid to the coupler in the test box.
4. Place the hearing aid and the reference microphone at the correct positions and close the lid.
5. Set the input at 65dBSPL. Press 'output curve only'. The machine will sweep through the frequencies. Print out the response curve.
6. Compare with the baseline frequency response curve recorded when the aid was new.
7. Harmonic distortion can be recorded at the same time. Harmonic distortion should be below 5 per cent in hearing aids for children.

References

Archbold, S. (1994) 'Monitoring Progress in Children at the Pre-verbal Stage', in McCormick, B. *et al.* (eds) *Cochlear Implants for Young Children.* London: Whurr Publishers.

Archbold, S. (1997) 'Cochlear Implants', in McCracken, W. and Laoide-Kemp, S. (eds) *Audiology in Education.* London: Whurr Publishers.

British Association of Teachers of the Deaf (1981, amended 1985) 'Audiological definitions and forms of recording audiometric information', *Journal of the British Association of Teachers of the Deaf* **5**, 3.

Bench, J. *et al.* (1979) 'A comparison of BKB sentence lists with other speech audiometric tests', *Australian Journal of Audiology* **1** (61), 61–66.

Berg, F. (1993) *Acoustics and Sound Systems in Schools.* San Diego: Singular Publishing Group.

Binder, J. *et al.* (1996) 'Functions of the left planum temporale in auditory and linguistic processing', *Brain* **119,** 1239–1247.

Boothroyd, A. (1968) *The Arthur Boothroyd (AB) Word Lists.* Manchester: University of Manchester.

Bouvet, D. (1990) *The Path to Language – Bilingual Education for Deaf Children.* Cleveland: Multilingual Matters.

British Society of Audiology (1986) 'Recommended procedure for taking an aural impression', *British Journal of Audiology* **20**, 315–316.

British Standards Institution (1980) *BS 5966: Specification for Audiometers.* London: British Standards Institution.

British Standards Institution (1984) *BS 6083: Methods for Measurement of Electroacoustical Characteristics.* London: British Standards Institution.

British Standards Institution (1988) *BS 2497: Part 5: Standard Reference Zero for the Calibration of Pure-Tone Audiometers.* London: British Standards Institution.

Carr, G. (1997) 'Development of Listening Skills', in McCracken, W. and Laoide-Kemp, S. (eds) *Audiology in Education.* London: Whurr Publishers.

Charlton, M. (1999) 'Implications of Literacy Strategy for Sign Language Pupils.' Unpublished MEd thesis. Leeds: Leeds University.

Fletcher, L. (1987) *A Language for Ben.* London: Human Horizon.

Flexer, C. (1999) *Facilitating Hearing and Listening in Young Children,* 2nd edn. San Diego: Singular Publishing Group.

Freeman, R. *et al.* (1981) *Can't Your Child Hear? A guide for those who care about deaf children.* London: Croom Helm.

Gregory, S. (1986) 'Advising the parents of young deaf children: Implications and assumptions', in Harris, J. (ed.) *Child Psychology in Action.* London: Croom Helm.

Hickson F. (1986) *The Manchester Picture Test (1984).* Manchester: Manchester University.

Johnson, C. D. *et al.* (1997) *Educational Audiology Handbook.* San Diego: Singular Publishing Group.

Kendall, D. C. (1954) 'Audiometry of young children', *Teacher of the Deaf* **L1**, 307.

Ling, D. and Ling, A. (1978) *Aural Rehabilitation: The Foundation of Verbal Learning in Hearing Impaired Childen.* Baltimore: University Park Press.

Lynas, W. *et al.* (1997) 'Supporting the education of deaf children in mainstream schools', *Deafness and Education* **21** (2).

Maltby, M. (1999) 'Winter deafness: A case study of a profoundly deaf child's additional hearing disability ', *Deafness and Education* **22** (1) 184–190.

Maltby, M. (2000) 'A new speech perception test for profoundly deaf children', *Deafness and Education International* **2** (2).

Marcshark, M. (1997) *Raising and Educating a Deaf Child.* Oxford: Oxford University Press.

McCormick, B. (1977) 'The toy test : An aid for screening the hearing of children above a mental age of two years', *Public Health* **91**, 67–69.

McCormick, B. (ed.) (1993) *Paediatric Audiometry 0–5 years* (2nd edn). London: Whurr Publishers.

McCracken, W. and Sutherland, H. (1991) *Deaf Ability not Disability.* Avon: Multilingual Matters.

Moores, D. and Meadows-Orlans, K. (eds) (1990) *Educational Aspects of Deafness.* Washington: Gallaudet University Press.

National Deaf Children's Society (1996) *Quality Standards in Paediatric Audiology. Vol. II: The audiological management of the child with permanent hearing loss.* London: National Deaf Children's Society.

Penhune, V. B. *et al.* (1999) 'The role of auditory cortex in retention of rhythmic patterns as studied in patients with temporal lobe removals including Hesch's gyrus', *Neuropsychologia* **37**, 315–331.

Reynell, J. and Huntley, M. (1985) *Reynell Development Language Scales.* Revised Edition. Windsor: NFER-Nelson.

Tate, M. (1994) *Principles of Hearing Aid Audiology.* London: Chapman and Hall. New edition in print: Maltby, M. (2001) *Principles of Hearing Aid Audiology* (2nd edn). London: Whurr Publishers.

Watson, T. J. (1957) 'Speech audiometry for children', in Ewings A. W. G. *Educational Guidance and the Deaf Child.* Manchester: Manchester University Press.

Watson, L. (1998) 'Oralism – current policy and practice', in Gregory S. *et al.* (eds) *Issues in Deafness.* London: David Fulton Publishers.

Webster, V. and Webster, A. (1997) *Raising Achievements in Hearing-impaired Pupils.* Bristol: Avec Designs Ltd.

Webster, V. and Wood, D. (1989) *Special Needs in Ordinary Schools: Children with Hearing Difficulties.* London: Cassell.

Wood, D. *et al.* (1986). *Teaching and Talking with Deaf Children.* Chichester: Wiley and Sons.

Index